Live a Little!

Also by Susan Love

Dr. Susan Love's Menopause and Hormone Book: Making Informed Choices (with Karen Lindsey)

Dr. Susan Love's Breast Book (with Karen Lindsey)

Also by Alice D. Domar

Be Happy Without Being Perfect: How to Worry Less and Enjoy Life More (with Alice Lesch Kelly)

Conquering Infertility: Dr. Alice Domar's Mind/Body Guide to Enhancing Fertility and Coping with Infertility (with Alice Lesch Kelly)

Self-Nurture: Learning to Care for Yourself as Effectively as You Care for Everyone Else (with Henry Dreher)

Healing Mind, Healthy Woman: Using the Mind-Body Connection to Manage Stress and Take Control of Your Life (with Henry Dreher)

Susan M. Love, M.D.,

Alice D. Domar, Ph.D.,

with Leigh Ann Hirschman

AND A LITTLE HELP FROM THE EXPERTS OF BEWELL

Live a Little!

Breaking the Rules
Won't Break
Your Health

Foreword by Nancy L. Snyderman, M.D.

 Three Rivers Press • New York

Published in the United States by Three Rivers Press, an imprint of the Crown
Publishing Group, a division of Random House, Inc., New York.
www.crownpublishing.com

Three Rivers Press and the Tugboat design are registered trademarks of Random
House, Inc.

Originally published in hardcover in slightly different form in the United States by
Crown Publishers, an imprint of the Crown Publishing Group, a division of Random
House, Inc., New York, in 2009.

Grateful acknowledgment is made to the following for permission to reprint previously
published material:

Bantam Books: Excerpts from *Mindless Eating: Why We Eat More Than We Think* by
Brian Wansink, copyright © 2006 by Brian Wansink. Reprinted by permission of
Bantam Books, a division of Random House, Inc.

Oxford University Press: "10-Year Risk Chart for Women" from "The Risk of
Death by Age, Sex, and Smoking Status in the United States" by Woloshin et al, in
Journal of the National Cancer Institute (vol. 100, issue 12). Reprinted by permission of
Oxford University Press.

Library of Congress Cataloging-in-Publication Data is available upon request.

ISBN 978-0-307-40943-0
eISBN 978-0-307-46243-5

Printed in the United States of America

Book design by Nicola Ferguson
Cover design by Jennifer O'Connor

10 9 8 7 6 5 4 3 2 1

First Paperback Edition

To Elizabeth Ann Browning:
You inspire us.

—SL and ADD

To Helen and Katie:
You help me live a lot.

—SL

To Dave, Sarah, and Katie:
You are my world.

—ADD

This book is designed to help you develop a balanced perspective on your health and make informed choices. It is not intended to replace advice from a health care professional who knows you personally. Before you make a significant decision about your health care, we urge you to get information from a variety of smart sources, listen to your own good sense, and talk the matter over with a doctor or other licensed health care provider who has earned your trust.

Contents

Foreword

This morning I had my nonfat Greek yogurt for breakfast, which is my usual start to the day. In fact, except for the days when I substitute a bowl of Cheerios in place of the yogurt, my breakfasts are not particularly daring. But it's always my hope that a good breakfast will lay the foundation for smart eating during the remainder of the day. I try to choose healthy foods, and that makes me feel good (and, as my friend Dr. Susan Love says, it also makes me feel morally righteous—even if only for a moment).

Now, based on what I've just told you and on the fact that I'm a doctor, you might think that I'm the paragon of good health. But you know by the title of this book that having a real life means not being perfect all the time. The goal is to be healthy—not a fanatic—and to live a little.

Living well starts with having concrete information, listening to that voice deep inside that tells you when things aren't quite right. It means living life to the . . . moderate.

Most of us do live somewhere in the middle, between the forty-yard lines. We are not meant to sacrifice all the time, nor gorge all the time. The end goal is to find that happy medium, then kick up our heels and, yes, live a little.

We all have our strengths (I don't smoke) and our weaknesses (Milk Duds). That's the point. Life is a balancing act. Life, our health, how we live day in and day out, is full of small and large decisions that have a bearing on our overall being.

Medicine is imprecise. It is a blend of art and science with one very, very important component—you. When it is at its best, modern (or for that matter, ancient) medicine is like a wagon wheel. You are the hub, and the doctors, nurses, pharmacists, healers, acupuncturists, massage therapists, and anyone else you rely on make up the spokes. It is made up of all these separate pieces, yet is also more than the sum of its parts. But it always, always should have you at its center.

One of the interesting things about that wheel, though, is that the spokes sometimes poke at one another. Doctors are like everyone else—we all have opinions and don't always agree with one another. That's good for you and, yes, sometimes confusing. It means that you don't have to take one person's opinion as gospel, but it also means that you have to do your homework.

Making health decisions for ourselves is like standing in the cereal aisle of a very big grocery store. There are so many choices that the simplest decision can be overwhelming. We think we know what to buy; we know how to read a label; we know the arguments about fat, protein, sugar, and fiber; we know what tastes good. So on one day we buy low-fat granola, and on another we find ourselves reaching for the Froot Loops. Such is life.

The same argument can be made for exercising (a word that I have come to believe is a four-letter word in disguise). Of course we know that exercise is good for us and keeps our HDL, the good cholesterol, up and makes our hearts and bones stronger. So on a good day, we take the steps and not the elevator. On other days, simply the idea of changing clothes and sweating sounds like just another chore.

Every day we make health decisions that affect our lives and the lives of our partners and children. We make these decisions based on our core beliefs, as well as from the bombardment of information streaming from television, print, radio, and the Web. As we get hit from all fronts we distill as much news as we can, balance it with a dose of common sense, and we may even feel the need to run everything by authority figures—our doctors.

And that's where things get interesting. What if one doctor sees things one way and another sees things differently? What are you supposed to do? Well . . . remember that wheel, where you are the hub? This is precisely where you read, listen, weigh the arguments, and put everything into the context of your life.

In this book two extraordinary women will take you through important issues that matter to all of us. They look at medicine from two vantage points. Dr. Alice Domar is a psychologist whose expertise is in stress and women's health. Dr. Susan Love sees life through the eyes of a surgeon and has written the bible on breast cancer. They are friends, colleagues, and bestselling authors who don't hesitate to speak their minds. They are passionate, brilliant, and along with their colleagues from BeWell, they cut through the science as well as the urban myths and talk openly and honestly about what we know in modern medicine, and what is pure conjecture.

They are not afraid to take on conventional wisdom, nor each other. And it is through their spirited debates that we learn. Through the lenses of two women who live and breathe medicine and research every day, we learn about the areas that concern us most regarding our health: stress, food, sleep, relationships, and more. In reading this book, you'll clearly see that doctors are patients, too.

There are a few things they agree on. There is no such thing as a safe cigarette, and Americans eat too much junk food. But venture beyond those subjects and see how the conversations change. What is the definition of being in shape? Do you really have to walk ten thousand steps a day? Is there merit to the annual physical examination? (Dr. Love says no, there isn't.) Ask Dr. Domar what constitutes a healthy relationship and it may not line up with Dr. Love's opinion. As for the optimal amount of sleep a woman should get . . . well, you'll have to open up the book for that one.

It is through their conversations and debates that we understand health. Life isn't always clear-cut and, yes, even the best experts can disagree. Where you will see consensus is in a moderate—a "pretty healthy"—approach to life. Again, the race is to the moderate, not the fringes.

We consume information differently and bring our own biases and interests to the table. And each of us brings a different genetic blueprint. But at the end of the day, medicine is best when it is wrapped in science and truth. That's the best any of us can do.

You can live your life without ever taking a bite of an Oreo and still get fat. You may be one of the lucky people who can smoke until you're ninety and not get cancer or emphysema. You never know. But why take the chance?

There are things you can control that really do affect the quality and length of your life. And there are things out of your control.

So what's the goal? What is a healthy life? I believe it is achieved by living your life the best way you know how. Forget about perfection. Perfection is elusive and will just make you crazy. Perfection is an imperfect goal. Being well, having fun along the way—living a little—that should be your new goal after reading this book.

So take inventory of your life. Look at the things that bring you joy and the things that bring you down. Consider what you really want to change. Think about your work and whether you are doing something that really excites and interests you. Be honest.

Follow your gut. Live your life well. Stop racing toward a goal that is not only impossible but also not much fun. Stay within those forty-yard lines, with some guidance along the way. Oh yeah, and don't forget that there's no reason to take it all so seriously. . . . Live a little!

Nancy L. Snyderman, M.D.
NBC News chief medical editor
Associate professor of Otolaryngology–University of Pennsylvania
Cofounder of BeWell.com

Chapter One

The Myth of Perfect Health

WHAT WOMAN CAN'T RATTLE OFF A LIST of to-do items for healthy living? Exercise for a healthy heart; train with weights to build muscle and bone; stretch to maintain mobility; eat meals that are carefully designed for good artery and bowel function; drink one glass of red wine daily to avoid heart disease; resist the temptation to drink *two* glasses of said wine to avoid breast cancer; get a full night's sleep to promote immune function; expose the skin to sunlight for ten minutes to absorb vitamin D, then immediately apply sunscreen to avoid skin cancer; relieve stress to strengthen the immune system; build a social support network to ward off Alzheimer's; book appointments with our mates for healthy sexual pleasure; and, of course, maintain a body mass index that falls exactly within the "healthy" range listed in every women's magazine.

And don't forget the Kegels.

This list is so impossible that it leaves most women either consumed with panic or doubled over with laughter. Yet if you have picked up this book, chances are you feel at least some obligation to follow what we'll call, with more than a dab of irony, the "health rules." The individual rules themselves may change with unsettling frequency—by the time you read this book, at least one of the rules we listed will probably be out of date—but one thing remains constant: Every time you turn on the television or read a magazine, you are bombarded with a highly specific set of dos and don'ts for staying healthy. Of course, you want to be healthy. And if you do get sick, you definitely don't want people to say, in an accusing tone, "She brought it on herself, you know, because she didn't eat enough broccoli." So you try.

But despite earnest efforts to follow these rules, you probably find it tough going. Maybe you've experienced the "what the hell" effect. *I've been "bad" and eaten a cookie. What the hell, I'll eat the whole bag.* Or: *There's no way I can exercise for sixty minutes every day. What the hell! I won't exercise at all.* Or perhaps you've done your level best to follow every piece of health advice and then been riddled with a sense of failure when you fell short. These experiences are common—all too common, we believe. The health rules, which are supposed to help us live longer and live better, have become a source of pressure, guilt, and stress. This is not a healthy situation.

We've written this book as a corrective to the narrowly laid-out health rules; in their place, we'll offer a more relaxed definition of both health and health habits. You might argue that we're exactly the kind of people who ought to be vigorously defending the conventional rules, not questioning them. And, yes, we've both devoted our lives to bettering the health of women. Susan is a breast cancer surgeon; the author of books about menopause and breast health;

and president of the Dr. Susan Love Research Foundation, an organization dedicated to ending breast cancer. Ali is a psychologist and author specializing in women's health; the head of the Domar Center for Mind/Body Health; the director of Mind/Body Services for Boston IVF; and an assistant professor of obstetrics, gynecology, and reproductive biology at Harvard Medical School. We're both part of BeWell, a team of health care professionals at the forefront of helping people live healthier lives.

In our jobs, we rarely encounter women who blithely ignore the health rules. Instead, we see women who are overwhelmed by them. So we decided to review the evidence for the health rules, sifting through piles of data—and guess what? We've come to believe what you have probably suspected all along: These rules are a little ridiculous. They are unrealistic, and, worse, their scientific foundation is often shaky. We're frustrated that you are made to feel guilty or hopeless when you can't conform to impractical and sometimes unsupported health guidelines. And we suspect that there are negative health consequences of worrying about your health all the time!

Great News: You Don't Have Total Control Over Your Health

We'd like to help you take on the health police—you know, those well-intentioned but literal-minded policy makers, television experts, magazine writers, personal trainers, and neighbors who make you feel like a lawbreaker every time you eat a gram of saturated fat. But to do this we have to address a difficult truth, which is that *we don't have total control over our health.* For too long, we've all been coached that if we follow certain health habits we will create a kind of protective bubble around our bodies, one that instantly deflects chronic diseases such as arthritis and hypertension. Pain-free and feeling great, we'll sally forth into old age with our bubbles intact, our bodies fortified by perfect diets and exercise regimens. The big nasties—cancer and heart disease—won't stand a chance against our flexible arteries and robust, well-regulated cells. Finally, at the age of 110, we'll say a moving good-bye to our loved ones and die peacefully in our sleep.

Sorry, but health doesn't work like this. Although there are habits clearly associated with premature disease, there are some determinants of illness and death that are beyond our control. (As the stress humorist and BeWell member Loretta LaRoche likes to say, those health nuts are going to be really surprised when they die of nothing.) All the yoga and stress reduction in the world might not be enough to counteract a genetic tendency toward, say, back pain. Or from being hit by that favorite morbid cliché of mothers everywhere, the city bus. On the other hand, we've all read the stories about one-hundred-year-old ladies who attribute their long lives to a diet of unfiltered cigarettes and butter. A true understanding of health takes into account the very real presence of luck, both bad and good.

But, you might ask, isn't there evidence showing that we can control our health by engaging in good habits? Well, if you poke at some of this evidence, you'll find it doesn't take long for that "total control" illusion to pop. For example, studies show that people who eat lots of fiber are less likely to develop heart disease than people who don't. What those studies don't tell us is whether the fiber-eating people live any longer. Do they have more years in which to enjoy life? Or do they simply die at the same age of an alternative disease, perhaps one that is not as mercifully quick and relatively painless as a heart attack? If th

better, or are the added years sp

sion? We simply don't know.

What we *do* know is that th

halfway believing that if you ea

in the proper way, you can escap

but death itself. This way of thin

orities: Instead of trying to be h

you squander your happiness in tl

Nortin Hadler, a professor of med ......y or North

Carolina, points out in his book *Worried Sick,* "The death rate is one

per person." We can't stop death, not even with oat bran.

Bleak news, yes. When you realize, though, that health is not under your total control, a lot of guilt and stress slide off your shoulders. It no longer feels as if your very life depends on how frantically you monitor your nutritional intake, exercise habits, and stress level. Better still, you can trade in your illusion of becoming perfectly healthy for something much more fun: being *pretty* healthy. Pretty Healthy means, first of all, that your health habits contribute to, not distract from, your enjoyment of life.

When you're Pretty Healthy, you live in such a way that you don't bring untimely disability or death upon yourself. You have sufficient supplies of energy, and you're free from obsession about the state of your body or your mind. Although you may suffer from illness now and then, or even develop a chronic health problem like osteoarthritis, you can still be Pretty Healthy if you take pleasure in life most of the time and possess the general sense that you can cope with the challenges that come your way.

There is good reason to think that pretty good health encompasses a much wider set of behaviors than we've been led to believe.

...ieve maximum vegetable consumption or get
...rs of sleep every night to "get it right."

...ere's the Evidence?

In the chapters that follow, we'll look at six areas—sleep, stress management, health screenings, exercise, nutrition, and personal relationships—that are the subject of many a health rule. Some of these
rules are based on excellent evidence. But many are not. Plenty are
based on scanty evidence or even bald corporate interest.

This is a sorry situation, but not a new one. Take a quick glimpse
back at the past decade of health journalism, and it's easy to think of
examples of health fads that rose on a wave of conjecture then re-
ceded when someone finally pointed out a lack of evidence. Just a
few years ago, you couldn't open a newspaper or magazine without
reading about the importance of drinking eight glasses of water a
day. Told they were in constant danger of dehydration, the women
of America (and many of the men, too) toted around giant bottles
of fancy, expensive water. Then the Institute of Medicine reviewed
the clinical literature and discovered there is absolutely no evidence
for the eight-glasses-of-water-a-day theory. It's hard to know how
the original myth got started, but it's impossible not to note that
bottled-water companies profited immensely.

Or take hormone replacement therapy (HRT). Actually, *don't*
take it. When Susan published books and articles that questioned
the widespread use of HRT for menopausal women—arguing in
particular that there was not enough evidence to draw conclusions
about either its benefits or its safety—she was attacked by both colleagues and the press. (One memorable article, published in the

New Yorker, was entitled "How Wrong Is Susan Love?") Then, in 2002, the first large-scale study of these treatments was halted before its completion, because clear evidence was already in: HRT not only fails to offer protection against heart disease and Alzheimer's, it increases the risk of breast cancer.

Now the time is ripe for examining other claims that are promoted as hard fact. Do we really need to eat a cup of blueberries every day? Must we exercise an hour daily, as the U.S. government announced in 2005? Is it necessary to have a baseline mammogram at age thirty-five? The answers are *no, no,* and *no!*

In the pages to come we are going to challenge the evidence for several health rules. But our point is not that we should give up on science entirely; instead, we should *lighten* up. The scientific method remains our best method for understanding what makes us healthy and what makes us sick. Sometimes the evidence is incomplete, *but that's okay, because you* are *capable of making good judgments based on incomplete evidence.* You do it every day when you make decisions about what to buy; the best route to work or school; and how to raise your children, if you've got them. Although the current medical evidence does not justify the kind of persnickety behaviors demanded by the health rules, you can still draw on a combination of the existing science and good judgment to determine which type of actions are probably Pretty Healthy. This rational process is what led us to the Pretty Healthy Zone.

The Pretty Healthy Zone

Over and over in our research, we've found that health habits tend to form U-shaped curves, with serious neglect on one end of the curve and obsession on the other. Both extremes are associated with poor health. If you are very overweight or very underweight, it's hard to be Pretty Healthy. If you have serious, prolonged, and uncontrolled levels of stress, or if you live in such a way as to avoid stress altogether, you're not Pretty Healthy. Women who never see the doctor are not Pretty Healthy, but neither are women who submit themselves to every screening the medical system can dream up. And so on.

But in between the extreme ends of the U-shaped curve is a very large area. We call this area the Pretty Healthy Zone, or PH Zone for short, because the behaviors here all seem to be conducive to a Pretty Healthy life. There are PH Zones for sleep, stress management, health screenings, exercise, nutrition, and healthy relationships. Each PH Zone encompasses a refreshingly wide variety of behaviors.

Take sleep. A good night's sleep is usually defined at somewhere between seven to eight hours of continuous rest. But Ali occasionally wakes up at night and can't get back to sleep for hours. Will she become sick as a result of missing sleep? Actually, Ali is well within the PH Zone for sleep. Most studies that connect sleep loss with illness have focused on people who get only four hours of sleep or less for many consecutive nights. Other, much larger studies show that people who get six or seven hours of sleep nightly live longer than those who get eight or more. They certainly don't appear to suffer from more disease as a result of their sleep patterns. And it appears that people can handle a certain amount of broken sleep. How else could we make it through college, new motherhood, or menopause?

Or let's look at exercise. The evidence for exercise is often overstated, leading many of us to worry that we will drop dead from

How We Studied the Studies

While writing this book we read hundreds of studies—about how much to sleep, what to eat, and what kind of exercise is most effective. We didn't take any of them at face value. Instead, we sifted through the details, constantly asking these questions:

• **What kind of study was it?** The most reliable studies are randomized, controlled trials (RCTs). The participants in an RCT are carefully screened and then randomly split into at least two groups: One gets the treatment that's being studied, and the other gets a placebo. Neither the participants nor the investigators know who is receiving the placebo and who gets the real deal. By "blinding" the scientists and subjects, the possibility of conscious or unconscious bias is significantly reduced.

But RCTs are expensive, difficult, expensive, time-consuming ... and, they cost a lot of money! There just isn't enough of the green stuff available for funding RCTs about most health questions. RCTs also pose obvious problems when it comes to studying long-term behavioral choices, such as exercise. How do you put a bunch of people in one group and say, "Be sure to exercise at a moderate to high intensity for exactly thirty minutes every day for the next ten years" and put a bunch of people in another group and say, "For the next ten years, stay totally sedentary—don't even run up a flight of stairs"?

When it's not possible to perform an RCT, scientists turn to observational studies. These studies track people's behavior over a period of time. Their habits are noted (often the subjects fill out questionnaires about a particular habit, such as how often they work out or whether they eat vegetables daily) as well as their illnesses, and then the study's investigators attempt to determine whether the two are connected. Observational studies can point out where two factors are significantly related, but one has

(continued)

to be careful. The relationship may be subtler. In one unnerving example, observational studies indicated that people with high blood levels of beta-carotene had lower rates of cancer, particularly lung cancer. For a while in the 1990s, smokers were popping beta-carotene supplements as if they were internal nicotine erasers. Then in 1994, the *New England Journal of Medicine* published the results of an RCT in which some people were given beta-carotene supplements and others were not. Not only did the beta-carotene group fail to show a reduced risk of cancer, the incidence of lung cancer in smokers who took the supplements shot up. Now smokers are advised *not* to take beta-carotene supplements.

Why this surprising result? Perhaps the people in the observational trial who had high blood levels of beta-carotene ate a lot of carrots instead of taking supplements. Perhaps they had less cancer because they also tended to eat a better diet in general, or maybe because they exercised more often. So when it comes to observational studies, things aren't always as they seem.

• **How many subjects were there?** No matter whether the study is an RCT or an observational trial, it's enlightening to see how many participants were involved. A study that tracks five people is usually less persuasive than a study that includes one hundred.

• **Was it performed on men or women? Humans or animals?** Our colleague Marianne Legato was among the first in the medical community to stand up and shout the news: *Women are different from men.* What is true for a man's body may not be true for a woman's. For example, it's now well known, thanks to Marianne, that 15 to 20 percent of women have very different heart attack symptoms than men do. And a study that shows an effect of, say, sleep loss on men may not tell us what sleep loss does to women. Studies performed on animals can be promising, but for obvious reasons they are inconclusive.

(continued)

> • **Was it conducted in an environment that mimics real life?** People's bodies may respond differently in a laboratory environment—where they may be nervous or excited—than in their daily lives.
>
> • **Who paid for it?** A study's source of funding may not be immediately apparent. Even though an industry group may not have directly financed a particular study, it may be paying the trial's investigators for other work, such as consulting. Most scientists try to remain unbiased—but that's hard to do when you know who signs your paycheck.

cancer or a heart attack if we don't get our daily workout. Not so, as we'll show you in the coming pages. But even though the link between exercise and good health is weaker than you've been told, we'll lay out a rational argument that exercise is nevertheless a *good bet* for staying healthy. With the knowledge that exercise is a Pretty Healthy habit, the next question is this: What if we can't get sixty minutes a day? What if we get thirty minutes? Twenty? Ten? Five? In the PH Zone for exercise, each of these options has a legitimate place, and you can use the evidence to help you decide which is most appropriate for you. The PH Zone also makes allowances for the ups and downs of a woman's life. Susan, for example, started an exercise regimen for the first time at age fifty. Does this make her less healthy than someone who has been exercising all her life? Probably not. As it turns out, middle age is right about the time when exercise becomes most important for maintaining vitality.

The PH Zones do not ask you to develop extremely difficult habits (such as sticking to a low-fat diet) or to maintain a precarious state of perfect balance (in which you experience exactly the right amount of stress, never too much or too little). Instead, the PH Zones allow you to relax in the knowledge that the normal variations we all experience—drinking mocha lattes; losing sleep; working late instead of exercising; and even occasionally eating Cheetos—can be part of a Pretty Healthy life. They also help you see that what you do on a particular day or week is less important than the patterns you create over the long term. Most health books try to convince you that unless you change your habits, you are on the fast track to disability and rot. We want you to realize that you are probably Pretty Healthy right now, just the way you are.

What If I'm Not in the PH Zone?

It happens. Even though the PH Zones are broad, there will be times when you find yourself perched high up on either end of the U-shaped curve, at one of the unhealthy extremes. Don't worry. The nice thing about the U-shaped curve is that it's a nice, easy slide down to center. After you've developed a more realistic attitude toward the health rules, you may find you're much less likely to have an all-or-nothing approach toward good habits. And we will help you reach your new, more moderate health goals, drawing on solid psychological techniques for making changes.

We'll also share our own experiences. As a working mother (Ali has two young daughters) and an empty nester (Susan has a daughter in college), we know a thing or two about how life's phases can sometimes pull us out of the PH Zone. We have personally struggled with the trade-offs between so-called ideal nutrition and the craving for a cheeseburger with fries; between spending enough time with our kids and getting enough sleep; between building our careers and managing stress. We have amassed a host of practical

A Side of Health

Throughout this book, we have asked the following BeWell Experts to contribute their knowledge and advice. We extend our deepest thanks to them all:

- Byllye Avery, B.A., M.Ed., founder of the National Black Women's Health Imperative and the Avery Institute for Social Change
- Elizabeth Browning, CEO of BeWell
- Christina (Chris) Economos, Ph.D., assistant professor of nutrition at Tufts University's Friedman School of Nutrition Science and Policy and associate director of the John Hancock Center for Physical Activity and Nutrition at Tufts University
- Laura Jana, M.D., pediatrician and the owner of Primrose School of Legacy
- Loretta LaRoche, stress management expert and humorist
- Marianne Legato, M.D., founder and director of the Partnership for Women's Health at Columbia University, founder of the Foundation for Gender-Specific Medicine, professor of clinical medicine at Columbia University, and adjunct professor of medicine at Johns Hopkins
- Miriam (Mim) Nelson, Ph.D., director of the John Hancock Center for Physical Activity and Nutrition and associate professor of nutrition at Tufts University's Friedman School of Nutrition Science and Policy
- Hope Ricciotti, M.D., associate professor of obstetrics, gynecology, and reproductive biology, Harvard Medical School

(continued)

- Pepper Schwartz, Ph.D., professor of sociology at the University of Washington in Seattle
- Nancy Snyderman, M.D., chief medical editor, NBC News
- Janet Taylor, M.D., psychiatrist in private practice

tips for working pretty good health into a packed schedule. At the same time, we like to think of ourselves as models for the Pretty Healthy philosophy that food cravings, exhaustion, and late nights are not necessarily bad or a cause for guilt. They are the inevitable, even desirable, companions of a full life.

To help make this point, we will also turn to our larger community of BeWell, a group of America's best and brightest medical experts who have joined forces to improve individual's well-being. BeWell Experts are some of the most respected names in their fields, but they are also real people, with real stress, real jobs, and real families. Throughout this book, we'll call on them for advice, ask them to debate controversial health topics, and reveal their personal strategies for staying Pretty Healthy. These are smart, compassionate, brave, and wickedly funny people, and we hope that their warmth and genuine desire to help you stay Pretty Healthy is something that remains with you long after you have finished this book.

Although the BeWell Experts don't agree with one another on every topic (for just one example, see our debate about the necessity of annual physicals on pages 82–84), we think you'll find our disagreements prove that there is no single, uniquely correct way to be healthy; there are many. But there is one opinion we all do share: True health isn't about devoting your hours to measuring fat grams, monitoring your heart rate, and going to bed early. A healthy life can and should be simple and enjoyable. If you aspire to be imperfectly—but happily—healthy, join us and read on.

Some people complain that health advice changes all the time, but we think it's great that scientists are constantly producing new studies. As more evidence about the topics in this book becomes available, we'll post our opinions on BeWell.com. Join us there!

Chapter Two

Sleep: When Lavender Sachets Don't Work

A LITTLE WHILE AGO, OUR FRIEND Anne had her first baby. Anne was talking to another mom at the park, and they agreed to meet for coffee. But when the woman asked for Anne's number, Anne drew a blank. Embarrassed, Anne admitted that she couldn't remember her own telephone number.

Her new friend's voice became compassionate but firm. "You're losing your memory," she said, "because the baby is keeping you up too much at night. If you don't get at least eight hours of uninterrupted sleep each night, your brain cells shrink and start to die."

Now there's a soothing thought: Motherhood causes brain death! As you can imagine, Anne found this piece of advice not only useless (who was going to nurse the baby while Anne got a good night's sleep?) but also upsetting. Was sleep loss really going to permanently harm her brain? Would staying awake with her crying newborn lead to Alzheimer's or worse? That night, the baby slept well, but Anne didn't. Despite her exhaustion, she was wide-eyed with worry over the damaging effects of *not* sleeping.

Sleep experts—and, as Anne discovered, just about everyone these days thinks they're an expert—love to tell us that sleep loss has dire consequences. *America is in a sleep crisis!* the reports shout. *Whereas we once averaged nine hours nightly, Americans now get less than seven. If you don't sleep at least eight straight hours at night, you'll get diabetes, you'll get fat, your immune system will shut down.* This drumbeat of pessimistic sleep news is a good way to catch our attention. (Did someone say "fat"?) It also sells a lot of sleeping pills. But is it based on solid science? Let's take a look.

The Eight-Hour Sleep Myth

We hear it all the time: *You need to get your eight straight.* Where did this belief come from? The study most often cited in support of the eight-hour claim was performed in 1993 by Thomas Wehr, M.D., at the National Institutes of Health in Bethesda, Maryland. In this study, sixteen healthy volunteers agreed to report to the lab in the late afternoon every day for four weeks. From 5 p.m. to 7 a.m., they spent fourteen consecutive hours in bed in a darkened room. At first, the volunteers slept an average of more than twelve hours a day. After a few weeks, most reduced their sleep time to somewhere between seven and a half and nine hours. Dr. Wehr concluded that the subjects slept a lot at first because they were typical sleep-deprived Americans who used the time to "catch up" on sleep and that the seven-and-a-half-to-nine-hour range was the optimal amount of sleep needed on a daily basis.

In a more recent but similar study at Harvard, seventeen women were given beds in dark, quiet rooms for twelve hours each night and four hours in the midday for three consecutive days. Most of the women slept much more on each of the three days than they usually did at home. When the study was published, the investigators announced that American women need more sleep than they get. The health news headlines repeated their conclusion.

There is another way to interpret these studies, however. Does the amount of sleep we get under ideal conditions—perfect silence and darkness, with abundant time to relax—reflect how much sleep we really *need*? Imagine if you were put under ideal *eating* conditions—say, in front of a banquet of delicious food—and told that you had to stay in the room for several hours with nothing to do but eat. How much would you eat? More than you usually would? More, perhaps, than you should? You can see where we're going with this analogy. These two sleep studies don't necessarily tell us how much sleep is necessary for good health. They indicate only how much people will sleep when there's nothing else to do. If you get less than this amount, are you really going to suffer terrible health consequences?

To answer this question, it's useful to look at studies that compare sleep amounts and mortality. In a study published in 2002 in the *Archives of General Psychiatry,* Daniel Kripke, M.D., tracked more than one million adults to find out which sleep durations corresponded to a longer life. He and his colleagues at the University of California at San Diego found that people who slept seven hours a night had the lowest rate of death over a six-year period. People who slept more than seven or less than five hours nightly had a greater risk of dying, though it is unclear whether this risk is due to the sleep habits themselves or to an underlying health problem, such as depression or heart disease.

This study doesn't tell any single person exactly how many hours of sleep is best for her own body, but it *is* reassuring, especially for women who are simply not capable of sleeping more than five, six, or seven hours a night. They can stop worrying about reaching the magic eight-hour number and know that the amount of sleep they're getting is not adversely affecting their health. Better still, this study suggests that we can all take a more relaxed and intuitive approach to sleep. According to Dr. Kripke's research (and a subsequent study at Harvard that backed up his results), sleep appears to follow the same bell curve as other health needs, including eating and exercise. As a general rule, people who exercise or eat either a great deal or very little are not as healthy as people whose habits fall somewhere in the middle range. Somewhere around seven hours of sleep is what most people get and what seems to be Pretty Healthy. Apparently our bodies know what's good for us after all.

You may ask why our current average of just under seven hours is so much lower than the nine hours people used to get a hundred years ago. It's a good question. One way to look at it is that we burn fewer calories these days than we used to, because we perform less physical activity. Maybe our sleep needs have changed as well. Or maybe we just slept more back then because there was little else to do after darkness fell.

Keep in mind that there are always normal variations on a bell curve and that you can't learn how much sleep you need from a book. You're the only person who knows what it's like to inhabit your body. If you've always needed eight to nine hours of sleep and feel terrible without it, use that information. Maybe all that sleep makes you more productive and happier than most people. Who's to say? Don't stumble around exhausted and miserable because a study tells you that seven hours is best. At the other end of the spectrum, if you feel great on six hours of sleep, go for it. Don't let the health headlines scare you into believing that you have a dreadful case of insomnia that must be artificially "cured." Enjoy your extra time awake. And when you are thinking about your sleep needs, remember that you don't have to be persnickety about getting the exact same number of hours every night. It's fine to get more sleep on some nights and less on others.

Another fact that gets lost in the sleep debate is that how much sleep you need—and how much sleep it's possible for you to get—can change over a lifetime. You may need a lot of sleep during adolescence, less in your twenties and thirties, and even less after menopause. During early motherhood and perimenopause, outside forces such as crying babies and hot flashes may limit how much sleep you get. But these phases don't last forever, and most women do not develop serious health problems as a result of going through them. (And Anne's "friend" had it all wrong. There's absolutely no evidence that sleep deprivation causes your brain cells to die. Some studies suggest that postpartum forgetfulness is caused not by sleep loss but hormonal ups and downs. Studies of adoptive parents—who suffer sleep loss but not hormonal changes—contradict this theory. Bottom line: Mothers get a free pass for forgetful behavior until their kids go to college.)

Won't We Get Sick, Fat, and Diabetic?

Sleep is more than an opportunity to take a break and rest our muscles. Rats who are totally deprived of sleep will die just as quickly as they would if they were starved of food. There is evidence that bodily healing and higher functions, such as the storage of facts and memories, take place during sleep. Of course, we also dream during sleep, and although we can't presume to tell you what purpose dreams serve, we know that our lives wouldn't be as interesting without them.

But considering that we spend about a quarter or a third of our lives asleep, scientists continue to have a pretty meager understanding of its purpose. Some researchers have approached this question by studying what happens when sleep is severely restricted. This is a legitimate method of scientific investigation, but unfortunately the media (and pharmaceutical companies) tend to draw far-reaching conclusions from small, focused studies. As a result, we're told that if we don't get those eight hours of sleep, we'll develop diabetes, or get sick a lot, or—perish the thought—gain weight.

For example, in one famous study, Eve Van Cauter, Ph.D., at the University of Chicago, put healthy young men onto a program of sleep restriction, allowing them only four hours of sleep per night. After eleven nights of short sleep, these men developed problems processing glucose. Many people have read this evidence to mean that sleep regulates our blood sugar and that sleep loss leads to diabetes. However, it's too early to reach such dramatic conclusions. For one, it's possible that the stress of taking part in a study, not the sleeplessness itself, produced the physiological changes. Second, the study looked only at young men. It doesn't tell us anything about how women or middle-aged subjects respond to sleep restriction. Finally, and most important, there are very few people who sleep only four hours per night for eleven nights in a row. What about people who cut their sleep short for just a few nights at a time? Or people who regularly sleep seven or six or five hours? The study also doesn't tell us what happens when people get more than four hours of sleep but less than the much-hyped requirement to get eight.

You may have heard reports that sleep-deprived people are more likely to suffer from weakened immune systems. In one study, people who normally sleep eight hours per night were asked to sleep only four hours—and blood tests afterward showed that their immune systems were suppressed. Does this mean that sleep regulates and repairs the immune system? Maybe, but it's hard to say how this study applies to the real world. Again, few of us who really need eight hours of sleep regularly try to get by on four. And again, the stress of the study—sleeping in a strange place and so on—may account for some of the immune changes. Finally, no one has shown that the kind of immune suppression produced in a petri dish leads to disease in humans.

For many women, the most distressing study about sleep produced headlines that read "Insomnia Makes You Fat." It's true that the Nurses' Health Study showed that women who sleep less than seven hours nightly gained more weight over a period of sixteen years than women who slept seven hours or more. But the weight gain was moderate. Women who slept five hours or less nightly gained an average of about five pounds more than women who slept for seven hours, and women who slept six hours gained about a pound and a half more. Again, the study points to seven hours—not eight!—as a good baseline. And it's not as if you will wake up one morning after a restless night and suddenly find yourself so big that you need to be hoisted out of your bed with a harness and crane. As always, the best course is to check in with yourself. Do you find yourself eating a lot more (especially chocolate, which contains caffeine) when you sleep less? Do you lose weight when you get more sleep? If so, you can decide on a rational course of action. If not, don't worry about it.

You will surely hear about many more studies that suggest unsavory consequences for women who don't sleep eight hours every night. It's important to weigh all the evidence carefully. As you consider the news you hear about sleep, remember to ask tough questions: Was this study conducted on people (not rats)? If so, how many people? Were they people like me (in terms of gender, age, and other factors)? Did the sleep-aid industry help fund the study? And, finally, remember that you can trust your body and your good judgment. If you are sleeping more or less than you need to, your body will give you signals. Listen to those signals, and you'll be fine.

Sleeping Through the Night

And what about quality of sleep—the idea that we need eight *straight* hours, uninterrupted by noise, worries, children, full bladders, or night sweats? A provocative 2007 study at Cornell University suggests that this ideal of "normal" continuous sleep may be a myth. This study, published in the *Journal of Sleep Research,* shows that most middle-aged adults fall asleep and stay asleep for several hours, then awaken for a few hours of quiet alertness, and then return to sleep until morning. Perhaps eight continuous hours of sleep is the norm only for younger adults, whose sleep has been more thoroughly studied. William Dement, M.D., a pioneer of sleep research, has always been careful to note that we know a lot about sleep in college students, who make handy subjects for science professors, but very little about what constitutes normal sleep in middle age. He likes to joke that his definition of a middle-aged person is someone who is too busy to participate in sleep experiments! (Fortunately, Cornell University found a few for this study.)

It may be that some adults sleep naturally and easily for long, continuous periods, and others don't—and that both patterns are

Pretty Healthy, as long you feel good during the day. Susan, for example, sleeps like a rock. She gets up in the middle of the night to go to the bathroom and doesn't even remember it in the morning. Ali follows the pattern in the Cornell study. Several nights a week, she falls asleep for about three and a half hours, wakes up for a few hours, and then goes back to sleep until morning. Before reading the study, she was worried that her wakeful nights would make her sick. Now she knows that most women her age follow her sleep pattern, which makes her feel better. "Okay," she thinks when she wakes up at night, "it's actually kind of nice to lie here peacefully, with no one making demands on me." If she starts to feel frustrated or worried, she breathes deeply or uses a relaxation technique called progressive muscle relaxation (described in detail on pages 44–45).

Even good sleepers will have times in their lives when plentiful, continuous sleep isn't an option. If you are growing a new family or a new business, if you are experiencing a creative surge on a favorite project, or if you are riding out the hormonal storms of perimenopause, sleep will be harder to come by. Assuming that your sleep loss isn't drastic and long-lasting, and that you don't drive when you're very sleepy, it won't kill you. Just do your best to get the sleep you can and try not to let the eight-hour sleep myth frighten you. It's not healthy to seriously deprive yourself of sleep, but it's also not healthy to become fearful and anxious just because you aren't carried off to eight hours of blissful sleep on the fluttering wings of butterflies—even though ad campaigns for sleeping pills suggest that you should be.

Speaking of commercials, one big problem we both have with advertisements for sleeping pills is that they suggest that sleep is something that should come easily—think of those glowing butterflies, alighting on sleepy suburban adults—without any discipline or

Quiz: Are You a Pretty Healthy Sleeper?

Instead of letting the eight-hour myth determine how much sleep you need, evaluate how you feel. If you get the right amount of sleep and you know it, feel free to skip this quiz. But if you suspect that

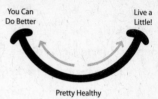

sleep loss is affecting the way you feel in the daytime, give it a try. For each symptom of sleep loss, circle the statement that most closely describes how you feel, then tally up your numbers and read about your score.

Sleep Loss Symptoms

Making Stupid Mistakes

0 points. You never make mistakes, especially when it comes to sleep. You never drink caffeine after noon, eat a big meal before bed, or miss your bedtime by even a few minutes.

1 point. Once in a while, you catch yourself putting your car keys in the refrigerator or making other odd errors, but your life isn't much affected by these rare trip-ups.

2 points. You frequently discover that you've done strange or silly things, and you're annoyed at how much time you have to spend correcting them.

3 points. You never catch yourself making stupid mistakes—but that's only because you're too tired to notice. Other people have to point them out to you before you realize what you've done.

(continued)

Irritability

0 points. The only time you feel irritable is when somebody interrupts your sleep.

1 point. You occasionally feel crabby, but you can successfully suppress the impulse to growl at your family or coworkers.

2 points. You're not nearly as nice as you used to be.

3 points. You're a bitch. Other people have commented about how irritable you are. Of course you're irritable, you think: No one else ever does anything right!

Forgetfulness

0 points. You like sleeping so much that you "forget" to set the alarm clock.

1 point. Your mind is like a steel trap. Mostly.

2 points. Last week you forgot a meeting or appointment.

3 points. Last week you forgot to pick up your kids from school. Twice.

Apathy/Lack of Motivation

0 points. You don't ever feel like going out with friends or letting the kids stay up late on the weekends because you might miss your 10 p.m. bedtime.

1 point. Sometimes you have to consciously summon up the desire to perform a task, but you can usually talk yourself into action.

2 points. Several times a week, you really struggle to get up and do what has to be done. Sometimes you decide to just let things slip.

3 points. You're too tired to care about anything. The house could be on fire or the kids could be cutting their hair with pinking shears,

(continued)

but you wouldn't mind—just as long as you don't have to get off the couch.

Yawning

0 points. You get eight or nine hours of sleep, but you still yawn a lot.

1 point. You yawn infrequently. When you do yawn, it's in the early afternoon or around bedtime.

2 points. Your boss says, "Am I boring you?" because you yawn during meetings.

3 points. Your husband says, "Am I boring you?" because you yawn during sex.

Lethargy

0 points. You wake up after a good night's sleep, creep downstairs in your jammies, eat some breakfast . . . and then you're ready for a nice nap.

1 point. You're a bundle of energy. All your friends scowl as you cheerfully wave at them as they stand in line at Starbucks.

2 points. Your level of physical fatigue interferes with some of your day-to-day activities.

3 points. You are so physically exhausted that every activity feels like a burden.

Inability to Concentrate

0 points. Your mind works more slowly than it used to. The more you sleep, the slower it gets.

1 point. There are some days when you're not as clearheaded as you used to be, but most of the time you're as sharp as ever.

(continued)

2 points. You find it very hard to concentrate at certain times of the day, especially the early afternoon.

3 points. It's hard for you to focus. Your mind wanders and you can't think clearly. If you don't write everything down, you are useless.

Depression

0 points. The only place you feel safe is under the covers.

1 point. You are cheerful and optimistic. You find lots of things to be happy about.

2 points. You have to push yourself to participate in life, but once you get going, you're okay.

3 points. You don't feel the same pleasure in life as you used to; the salt has lost its savor. You feel hopeless about the future.

Scoring

0–5 points: For one reason or another, you seem to be getting too much sleep. You definitely lack energy. Try going to bed a little later, waking up a little earlier, and getting more exercise. If you still feel lethargic or obsessed with sleep, check in with your doctor. You may have an underlying condition that's causing you to feel sleepy all the time.

6–11 points: Although you have occasional symptoms of sleep loss, you tend to get the right amount of sleep for your needs. Congratulations . . . you're right in the middle of the PH Zone.

12–17 points: Your body and mind are feeling the wear and tear of sleep loss. Never mind what the studies say about sleep requirements—your body is telling you that you're not getting enough.

18–24 points: Your exhaustion affects you both physically and psychologically. You can't be Pretty Healthy when you're this tired. Read on for suggestions that will improve your sleep.

effort. But for most of us, effortless sleep is a relic of childhood, in the same category as the endless summer. Like it or not, some people have to put a good night's sleep on their to-do list. It's not necessarily going to happen naturally. In the rest of this chapter, we'll suggest ways you can make better sleep happen. Start with the quiz, which will help you check in with your body so you can decide if you need more sleep than you're currently getting.

Serious Sleeplessness: When to Worry

Sleeplessness happens. Problems with sleep, however, can sometimes be caused by medical conditions such as sleep apnea, restless legs, hypertension, thyroid problems, depression, anxiety, or heart disease. If you have *new* and *unexplained* changes to your sleep habits—suddenly sleeping much less or much more than usual—and if these changes last more than two weeks—get checked out by a doctor.

A Pretty Good Night's Sleep

If you're not getting as much sleep as your body needs, the best place to start is with your sleep habits. You may already know some of the basic good sleep habits—cutting off your caffeine supply in the afternoon, avoiding alcohol in the evening, going to bed at the same time each night—but most of us hate to use them. Unfortunately, they work!

Why are good sleep habits so difficult? Probably because so much of contemporary life emphasizes nighttime stimulation and makes the master bedroom the hub of home activity. (We're waiting for beds that come equipped with coffee cup holders. Why not? Cars, strollers, and bicycles already have them.) Going against such strong cultural tendencies is doable, but it's an uphill battle. So instead of asking you to make a bunch of behavioral changes all at once, we suggest taking baby steps toward better sleep behaviors. Start with little, easy changes, like these:

- Keep your bedroom cooler. Open a window or, if it's noisy outside, turn down the thermostat.
- Wear light clothes to bed and use light bedcovers.
- Watch television, work, and read somewhere other than your bed.
- Don't eat a big meal just before bedtime.

If, after a few days, your sleep still needs improvement, progress to these steps, adding them one at a time:

- Expose yourself to thirty minutes of bright sunlight every day, whether outside or near a window.
- Make four o'clock in the afternoon your cutoff time for caffeine (the average person needs four to six hours to fully metabolize the drug).
- Limit yourself to one glass of alcohol in the evening. (Alcohol can help you fall asleep faster, but it disrupts your sleep later on.)
- Exercise during the day to promote better sleep. (But don't exercise just before bed, because your body temperature will be too high to induce sleep.)
- Avoid disturbing books or television shows before bed, including the news.

Then, if you need to, move on to the hard stuff:

- Go to sleep and wake up at the same time every day.
- Get out of bed when you can't sleep.

The last item—getting out of bed when insomnia strikes—is tough for most of us. If the sleep fairy arrives, we want to be there! But this

---

From the Trenches...

I think sleep is very important. I like to get at least eight to ten hours. If the people in my family would let me, I'd go to bed at 7 p.m. I've always been like this. I start winding down at five in the evening, and I don't really want to do much after that.

So I don't have any trouble falling asleep at night, but what happens as we get older (I'm in my seventies) is that we have to get up to go to the bathroom. I've heard that you wake up first and *then* you have to go to the bathroom, but it feels the other way around to me. I think I wake up because my bladder starts screaming. Then I go to the bathroom, and when I come back I have trouble falling asleep. Sometimes I will lie there for hours and not go back to sleep. I've tried all the things you're supposed to do: I don't look at the clock. I don't turn on all the lights. One thing that does work for me is to get up and read or work on the computer. It puts me to sleep. If I'm in a hotel room, I turn on the TV. Nothing puts me to sleep like CNN and the constant repetition of the same news.

So I'm struggling, but I've noticed that since I started exercising I'm more able to fall back asleep when I wake up at night. That's good, but I hate that the answer to everything is diet and exercise!

—*Byllye Avery*

advice is based on terrific evidence. In a controlled study performed at Duke University Medical Center, this approach (which included other good sleep habits, such as standardized wake and bed times), reduced sleep fragmentation by 50 percent. This means that the time it took the subject to get back to sleep after waking up at night was cut in half, and so were the number of night wakings. That's a better response than many sleep medications can claim, and there are no side effects. The idea is that you want to condition your body to associate your bed with sleeping, not with wakefulness. This conditioning takes time, so the technique might not work on the very first night. You may experience a few frustrating nights before you have a breakthrough, and that's what makes it so hard for people.

Don't be too angry with yourself if it takes a while to change your habits. As a species, we're much better at small changes than big ones. But the experience of a small success tends to inspire us toward even greater improvement.

Of course, good sleep habits aren't always enough. All the sleep hygiene in the world won't protect your sleep from a squalling baby or crushing work deadlines. We're always annoyed by so-called sleep tips that have nothing to do with reality, such as these:

Tuck a lavender sachet under your pillow. We'll admit that lavender is soothing, but how will it keep your children from running into your bedroom at 3 a.m.?

Take a nap. Hmmm . . . not sure that would go over well at the office.

Don't stay up late watching TV. This seems unfair. After sixteen straight hours of working, caregiving, and running errands, women aren't allowed to unwind in front of *The Daily Show*?

Instead, let's look at some real obstacles to women's sleep and come up with some realistic solutions. Because a lot of sleep deprivation begins with motherhood, we'll start there. But if you don't have children or if your kids don't keep you awake at night, you can go directly to the section that addresses your concerns.

Motherhood

A woman loses an average of 740 hours of sleep in the year after her baby is born. These sleepless nights aren't all bad. During the newborn period, some women learn to cherish the time alone with their babies in the quiet of the night. Others think of this sleepless time as a rite of passage into a new stage of adulthood. These positive thoughts can help a mother adapt to new physical and emotional stresses.

At the same time, we shouldn't lose perspective. The newborn period wasn't meant to last for eighteen years. It's normal to lose some sleep when your kids are sick, scared, or going through a time of adjustment, but if you are constantly exhausted because your children keep you awake night after night, it's your job to mend the family sleep patterns. Think about how *your* parents managed. In our families, the door to the master bedroom was closed at night, and God help you if you knocked on it. Ali's appendix ruptured one night when she was twenty-three and home from graduate school—and even at that age and in her situation, she was hesitant to wake her parents and get help! Now things are very different. Most of us sleep with our bedroom door open, and the children know that there's a standing invitation to climb into their parents' bed.

Laura Jana, a pediatrician and owner of a child-care center, believes that we fool ourselves into thinking it's good for our children to rely on us so much at night:

Being a pediatrician doesn't prepare you for having kids of your own. It's much easier to see them in the office than to live with them—and sleep with them. Now that I have my own children, I talk to parents a lot about sleep. I ask them: Do you feel good when your kids are waking you up at night? Of course, the parents admit that they feel awful when they don't sleep. My belief is that the kids don't feel any better. There's no reason to think that endless nights of interrupted sleep make you miserable but make your baby or pre-schooler feel great.

A technique called "controlled crying" is a compassionate but firm way to teach babies and children how to sleep. Entire books have been devoted to controlled crying—we recommend both *Solve Your Child's Sleep Problems* by Richard Ferber, M.D., and *Sleeping Through the Night* by Jodi Mindell, Ph.D.—but here are the basics:

1. Use this technique only for babies and children who are at least six months old and in good health.

2. Make sure the child has a comfortable, dark, quiet sleeping environment.

3. Put the baby in the crib (or tuck an older child into bed). Say good night.

4. Leave the room.

5. If the child protests, don't dash right back in. Wait five minutes and then briefly return to reassure the child. Don't pick the child up, and spend no more than a minute in the room.

6. Wait again for the child to settle down. Remain outside the room, this time for ten minutes, before going in to briefly reassure the child.

7. Continue this pattern as long as necessary, making each interval of time outside the room longer. The child will know that you

haven't abandoned him or her but will also understand that crying won't bring you back quickly.

Most children take about an hour to fall asleep on their own the first time. It's natural to want to stop the process and rescue your crying child. But when parents are consistent, most children will fall asleep by themselves without protesting by the third night. Most children who learn to fall asleep on their own at the beginning of the evening will soon learn to sleep through the night without your help—but if yours doesn't, you can use the controlled crying technique for nighttime wakings as well.

If you are trying to teach a mobile toddler to sleep through the night alone, you may have to continually steer him or her back to bed without granting too much of your attention or emotion. This can be a difficult, dull, exhausting process, but in the long run you'll both sleep better.

When children are old enough to talk and reason, other strategies are more useful. Ali's daughter Katie is seven years old and sometimes wakes Ali up at night, just to reassure herself that Mom's still there. (Ali's cousin Katherine calls this "refueling.") Katie, relieved, goes right back to sleep after Ali steers her back to bed—but Ali, once awakened, may be up for hours. To address this problem in a positive manner, Ali and her older daughter made up a star chart for Katie. For every night Katie went through the night by herself, she received a star, and seven stars in a row entitled her to a new Webkinz stuffed animal. (In case you're not spending time with the twelve-and-under crowd, Webkinz are stuffed animals with a virtual life on the Internet.) Katie's nighttime trips stopped immediately and for several months the behavior seemed to have sunk in—and then it slowly wore off again.

It's clearly time for Ali to do another star chart, because waking up so much at night is starting to get frustrating for her. And if that doesn't work, there will eventually have to be repercussions, but rewarding good behavior is usually far more effective than punishing the behavior you want to change.

Of course, sleep loss doesn't end when your child starts to sleep through the night. You have sickness, nightmares, and bed-wetting ahead of you. Then they start driving and dating—and suddenly *you* are too scared to sleep.

As a mother, you have to walk a fine line. You are hardwired to listen for trouble at night and to protect your kids, so a certain amount of sleep loss comes with the territory. But you also have to use judgment about how quickly you leap out of bed to help your children and how much you worry. A good example comes from Elizabeth Browning, BeWell's CEO. When her son Ian began to drive, she stopped sleeping. She stayed awake imagining the worst— wild parties, drunk driving, and accidents.

Then Ian said to his mother, "If I'm fifteen minutes late, why do I have to be wrapped around a telephone pole? Why can't I just be having a good time?"

When Ian pulled the car out of the driveway the next weekend, Elizabeth closed her eyes and, instead of panicking, imagined him having fun with his friends. She woke up when he came home—and then sank gratefully back to sleep.

Stealing from Sleep to Relax

Ali was meeting with a new patient one day. They had been talking for a while when Ali asked a routine question: How much sleep do you get?

"Oh, about five or six hours a night," said the woman. "I'm tired all the time."

"If you're tired all the time, five or six hours of sleep isn't enough for you," Ali said. She explained to her patient that if she could get to a point where she wasn't so tired, her stress levels would go down considerably. The woman would feel a lot better—and maybe not even need to see a therapist anymore.

To start brainstorming about how the patient could get more sleep, Ali asked her what time she woke up in the morning.

"The kids wake up at six every morning," the woman said, wearily.

Six a.m. is a brutal but typical wake-up time for young children, who tend to rise with the sun. (Until, of course, they start school and have to catch an early morning bus. *Then* they want to sleep in late.)

"So, counting backward," said Ali, "if you want to try for seven hours of sleep you need to have the lights out at eleven p.m."

"I can't do that!" the woman protested. "By the time I make dinner and stuff the children into bed it's nine o'clock. That's when I do laundry, answer e-mail, and get to talk to my husband. And after *that,* I really want some time for myself. So I watch television for a while. But then I'm kind of revved up, so I don't fall asleep until midnight or one o'clock in the morning."

The National Sleep Foundation's 2007 "Sleep in America" poll shows that 85 percent of women who spend less than six hours in bed at night also stay up late watching television. This has led many sleep advocates to tell us that if we'd just kick the TV habit, we'd get more sleep. There's some truth to this, but blaming late-night television masks a legitimate complaint of Ali's patient and other women: The late evening is the only time that many can carve out for themselves to relax. It just happens that women are so tired that watching television is often the way they choose to wind down.

You deserve to relax and nurture yourself without robbing your sleep bank. This means you'll have to do some creative rearranging during the day and early evening. Here are some suggestions for easing the time crunch, so that you'll have time for both sleep *and* self-nurture.

• **Write down all the things you want to accomplish during the day, and ask yourself: How can I do two of them at one time?** Susan listens to books on tape or medical research material while she runs. Or you can exercise with your spouse or partner, which gives you a chance to catch up without the world bearing down on you. Or you can invite a friend over for a chat while you declutter your kitchen.

• **If you work, exercise during half of your lunch hour** (if you're lucky enough to get an entire hour) instead of in the morning or evening. Use the extra time to sleep.

• **Delegate.** Most of us vastly underestimate how much our spouses, children, or elderly live-in parents can help us. Direct them toward a specific task: washing vegetables, folding laundry, or putting dishes into the dishwasher. This can free up more time for you in the evening.

• **Realize that there's nothing wrong with not spending every minute "being productive."** For example, you can read a book after dinner while your kids do their homework; you don't have to hover over them. Then you won't have to squeeze in your downtime late at night.

• **Reassess your kids' bedtime.** Adjust it according to your child's mood when he or she wakes up in the morning. Sleep needs vary, but preschoolers who wake at the crack of dawn probably need to be in bed earlier than nine o'clock. So make sure that our society's preference for activity over sleep hasn't also deprived your children of needed rest time. When kids get all the sleep they need, they'll be more focused and less cranky during the day, *and* you'll have more time for yourself in the evening. Use your judgment here. Don't force an artificially early bedtime onto wide-awake kids just because you're ready for some adult time.

· **Limit your children's extracurricular activities.** We wish there were a federal law mandating that kids can be scheduled for no more than two activities per season. There's not a single child psychologist or college admissions officer who will tell you that trumpet lessons for a five-year-old are more important than unstructured time to play. The side benefits are that all the members of your family will be more likely to have dinner together and you'll also get to bed earlier.

· **Schedule time for yourself every day.** Your body and mind crave time to relax and unwind. Don't create a schedule that ignores this need; instead, guide yourself or your family into a routine that frees you up at the same time every night, for example, from 9 to 10 p.m.

· **Choose self-nurturing activities thoughtfully.** You can spend two hours staring glassy-eyed at a television show you don't even like—or maybe you could take one hour to thoroughly enjoy a great program you've recorded. Or perhaps reading, meditating, or writing in a journal would be more renewing for you. Also, be aware that some TV shows, like crime dramas or the evening news, are highly stimulating and can make it harder for you to fall asleep.

From the Trenches . . .

Unlike many people with sleep problems, I have no trouble sleeping. I can sleep on planes before takeoff. Last night I fell asleep during the opening act for a rock concert! When I hit the bed, I am asleep in minutes. Sometimes I wake up so groggy that all I can do is think about getting back into bed, and it takes a very long time before I really feel awake.

What is my problem? I put too much in a day—and I can't stop. I get up early so that I can get more meetings and work in. I start cleaning up my life when I get home, no matter what time that is. I might clean a particularly disgusting closet that has been annoying me, or realize that a deadline is coming closer and finish an article. I am not above going over unread e-mail and attacking it, only to look up to notice that it is 2 a.m. Friends, horrified, write me letters about the time the e-mail was written. Where did the time go? The only way I notice is that I am nodding off. Dumb and dumber.

My body wants more sleep than it's getting. So what am I doing to combat my pattern? Well, the first thing is to treat it seriously. I am not eccentric and I am not hardworking, although these are compliments I used to excuse staying up late. Now I tell myself that I am being self-destructive . . . and I have to cut it out.

Second, I do not allow myself the luxury of things that seduce me to stay up longer. I am making and enforcing a rule not to answer e-mail in the wee hours of the morning. No TV after ten unless it's something really special and a treat. I sleep a half hour longer in the morning and meditate a bit before starting my day.

Have I licked the problem? No. It's a longtime habit and it's hard to break. But my motto to myself is "baby steps"—meaning that one small change at a time is doable and progress to be proud of. My goal is to get eight hours of sleep at least a couple nights a week. What am I at? About six. What is not unusual for me? Four or five. Recently, I've had whole weeks where I've had seven. I am on my way to my goal!

—*Pepper Schwartz*

Work and Chores

Women who want more sleep often come up against a basic fact of American life: We work a lot. If you work for money, you have probably spent your share of evenings working from a laptop or Black-Berry in bed. Even if you don't bring home a paycheck, you may still have more work to do than your mother did, because the pressure on stay-at-home women has also increased. We are supposed to cultivate a flawless but unique personal style that is reflected in our homes, hair, and clothes; work intensely with children on academics and activities; and shun our mothers' Hamburger Helper for elegantly presented organic meals inspired by the professional chefs on TV. Sometimes it's exciting to stretch the boundaries of what you can comfortably achieve in a day—and sometimes it's just not. This is especially true if you are so tired you can no longer enjoy your accomplishments.

It may not be in your power to significantly reduce your load at the office, especially if your boss believes that insomnia is a virtue. You do have control over your attitude toward work, however, and that can change how much work you do at night. Nancy Snyderman, who is chief medical editor for NBC News as well as a practicing surgeon, knows a little about letting go of the warrior mind-set. "All surgeons go through a stage where they brag about how little sleep they get. I did it, too. It makes you feel as if you're in an elite club," she says. "But everyone eventually gets to a point where they realize that sleep deprivation is not working for them." And try not to feel pressured by coworkers or neighbors who boastfully say things like "I'm so busy!" or "It's only June and I'm booked through December!" They may be exaggerating—or they may derive their self-worth by being busy all the time. Either way, these people probably aren't Pretty Healthy role models.

Which Came First, Insomnia or Red Bull?

For most people, there's nothing wrong with drinking a couple cups of coffee every day. But if insomnia or interrupted sleep is making you crazy, find out whether caffeine is the cure for your exhaustion, or its cause.

You expect Red Bull and other "energy" drinks to have lots of caffeine, but the caffeine content of some foods and beverages can be surprising. A grande cup of Starbucks coffee contains 372 milligrams of caffeine, which is more than three times what you'd get in a home-brewed cup. No wonder people enjoy hanging out at coffee shops—they're *flying* from all the caffeine. Chocolate, mocha ice cream, coffee yogurt, iced teas, colas, Barq's root beer, and Sunkist orange soda are also significant sources of caffeine. If you consume any of these caffeine sources after four o'clock in the afternoon, you might feel their effects when you try to sleep. Some people take even longer to process caffeine and can't touch coffee any later than noon. And some of us use caffeine to temporarily mask how desperately sleepy we really are. When the coffee high passes, we crash—and wonder why we feel so crabby and out of control.

Sleep and Stress

Sometimes what might be a few hours of temporary insomnia can snowball into something bigger. You have trouble sleeping—and then you worry about the consequences of not sleeping, so you sleep even less. Pharmaceutical companies prey on these fears by suggesting that if you don't get eight hours of sleep every night, you will suffer immediate and devastating sickness. Sleep then becomes a performance problem that perpetuates itself, and you can find yourself dreading night's arrival.

Stress-reducing techniques can head off this cycle. Let's face it: Turning over your worries in your mind at night can be very tempting. It almost feels good, in a biting-on-a-canker-sore kind of way. Sometimes you need another focal point to replace your mental worry list. Meditation, focused breathing, and visualization are all great for this purpose. When you are worried because you have more work than you think you can accomplish, get out of bed and write down your worries. Getting your fears down on paper helps (then you won't have to worry that you'll forget what to worry about) and chances are that you'll realize things aren't as bad as they seem. You've been pitched into overwhelming times before, and you've pulled through.

Another technique, called progressive muscle relaxation (PMR), has repeatedly been proven to help people fall asleep faster at bedtime and—this part is crucial—to help them return to sleep after waking in the middle of the night. Don't let PMR's medical-sounding name put you off. The exercise simply asks you to squeeze and release muscle groups in your body, starting with your head and moving down. It's very pleasant. Here's how to do it:

• Lie on your back, breathing deeply. You can stay in bed or move to the couch, or even the floor. (PMR is also a great tool for general stress reduction; if you are using it to chill out but don't want to fall asleep, try sitting in a chair or other comfortable spot.)

• Tense the muscles of your forehead. Try to bring your eyebrows as close together as possible. Imagine that you're scrunching those forehead muscles—really go at it. After a few seconds, release the muscles and completely relax your scalp. Imagine your muscles feeling warm, relaxed, and happy.

• Repeat this sequence of tensing, holding, and releasing as you move down your body. (This is the "progressive" part, like a progressive dinner that moves from house to house.) Travel from your scalp to your face, jaw, neck and throat, shoulders, hands, upper back, abdomen, pelvis, thighs, knees, lower legs, ankles, and feet.

• If you like, add a different visual or sensory dimension. Think of your muscles becoming soft and pliant, or imagine a color streaming into your relaxed body. Do you like healing blue, or gently warming red?

No matter how you perform PMR, you may discover that you've been holding tension in your body without even realizing it. When you're done, your body should feel relaxed and heavy.

Of course, stress reduction techniques aren't magic, and even if you are a Buddhist monk there will still be nights when you are too tense to sleep. When this happens, say to yourself, "I guess I'm having a no-sleep night. It's no big deal. This happens to everyone now and then." If you're a mother, you can say, "I survived sleep loss when my kids were newborns, and I will survive it now." You can get up and do something you enjoy, or maybe just lie in bed and, like Ali, appreciate having time to think quietly and freely. Note, though, that if you have frequent insomnia, you shouldn't make a habit of lying in bed awake. Your body will start to associate the bed with wakefulness, which will make it even harder to sleep on subsequent nights. Move to the couch or a chair instead.

When you are under extreme pressure, your body can send you distress signals, including headaches, joint pain, and insomnia. Unless there is an organic reason you're not sleeping well (see page 30), maybe your body is asking you to change your behavior. Instead of saying, "Oh no, I'm not sleeping," you can try saying, "What's the problem? What am I worried about?" Maybe you need to adjust your life to reduce stress or give yourself more time to wind down before bed. Maybe there's a serious problem that is calling out for your attention. Identify the problem and, if possible, try to work through it. If it's not a problem you can solve—say, your father has Alzheimer's—try to manage your *reaction* to the problem through exercise, meditation, and other stress management techniques.

But as much as we believe in gentle, commonsense treatments, we also know that some problems are too big for self-care alone. Long-term stressful situations, such as divorce or serious debt, can lead to long-term sleep disruption. You can't medicate these problems away, but when stress continually overpowers your ability to sleep, it's not wrong or weak to take sleep medications. After Ali's mother died, her grief manifested itself as anxiety. After a couple of sleepless weeks, she ended up taking Ambien for a few weeks to get her body back into a normal sleep-wake cycle. She now knows that if something is going on in her life that severely disrupts her sleep and can't be resolved through gentler means, Ambien will click her back into normality. In a Pretty Healthy life, sleep medications can have their place.

The Skinny on Sleeping Pills

When insomnia hits, your first line of defense should be lifestyle changes, which are described in detail on pages 30–32. It's always healthier to rely on your own resources rather than a pill. But sometimes sleep medications can stop a downward spiral of sleeplessness and set you right again. In those cases, which drugs are best?

We've all heard horror stories about the old-style sleep medications that caused addiction, withdrawal, and groggy hangovers. The new sleep medications, including zolpidem (Ambien), ramelteon (Rozerem), and eszopiclone (Lunesta), are much better. They do not cause physical addiction and are good for pulling you through a rough patch (no longer than a few months). However, these drugs all have side effects, including psychological dependence, so don't use them on a continuous basis.

Melatonin, a hormone that plays a key role in the sleep-wake cycle, is not the miracle sleep drug that it was once made out to be. But it appears to be safe for use in the short term and may be useful for people who have trouble falling asleep at bedtime (as opposed to people who wake up in the middle of the night). It may also be good for shift workers, world travelers, and others who need to reset their biological clocks in order to sleep. Susan uses melatonin when she travels overseas; however, Nancy Snyderman says that she has too strong a response to the supplement. "I took it once after a trip and lost a whole day of my life," she says. So you may have to experiment a little before you find the sleep aid that's best for you.

If you want to try alternative medicine for better sleep, you can try acupuncture, chamomile, or valerian. They are all safe for most people to try, but good clinical trials have yet to prove their effectiveness. Acupuncture and chamomile are also pleasantly relaxing. The same cannot be said for valerian, which smells like old socks, so try mixing it with a strong-flavored drink, such as pineapple juice, that will (somewhat) mask the odor. Avoid kava kava, because there have been reports of liver failure following its use.

Hormonal Changes

Simply put, women need less sleep as they get older. Hot flashes and night sweats especially affect a woman's sleep as she encounters perimenopause. During perimenopause, your body is comfortable

From the Trenches...

I don't sleep much. Many other postmenopausal women also have trouble sleeping. Instead of joining the "sweat and fret club," whose members wake up at 2 a.m., staring into the dark and wondering why they can't sleep, relax and say, "Well, my nights are not what they were before menopause." Maybe postmenopausal sleep loss is an evolutionary attempt to get you to enjoy more of the time you have left!

—*Marianne Legato*

only within a fairly narrow range of temperatures—meaning that you can feel freezing even when it's just a little chilly outside and that you start to sweat during a brief but hot shower. Susan, a former Boston resident now living in Los Angeles, laughs about how people in the Northeast love to sleep in their flannel pajamas, tucked under down comforters. But if you're warm and cozy when you go to bed during perimenopause, you can easily overshoot that new, narrow temperature range and wake up soaked with sweat. Wickaway clothes, like the ones available for exercise, are good because they don't give you the clammy feeling you get with wet cotton. Go to bed just on the edge of being too cold; you'll have a much better chance of sleeping through the night. If you make these changes but hot flashes continue to seriously disturb your sleep, consider taking estrogen for a limited period of time.

Hot flashes are not the only cause of sleep problems during perimenopause and menopause—though it is not clear exactly what causes sleep difficulties during this time of life. When nothing else works, short-term use of estrogen or micronized progesterone supplements often resolve insomnia very quickly. But many women instinctively want to address menopausal symptoms through gentle means. This is a wise first course of action for sleep problems at any stage of life.

WHEN YOU ARE HAVING TROUBLE sleeping, no matter what the reason, it's good to know that most sleep problems last for only a short time. One of Dr. Kripke's studies at the University of California at San Diego shows that although people may have short amounts of sleep on a particular night, or even for a week's worth of nights, the number of sleep hours they get over the course of the year usually averages out to a normal amount. So try to take the long view. Instead of focusing on how little sleep you had last night or last week, concentrate on the pattern that evolves over a month or a year. This positive outlook might just help you wind down . . . and finally get some sleep.

Chapter Three

The Stress Test: How Much Is Too Much?

STRESS IS GOOD. STRESS IS *great*. If you restrict your highs and lows in an attempt to reduce stress, you won't be healthier. You'll just be bored. And boredom is definitely not good for you, because monotony is death.

If you don't believe that stress is desirable, try thinking of someone you know who is absolutely carefree. We'll bet that this person is not a radiantly healthy, energetic adult. Most likely, it's someone under the age of twelve . . . or a person in pathological denial. No, you definitely don't want to be *that* mellow. The discomfort of stress is a sign that you are getting down in the trenches and wrestling with life's tough problems head-on. Good for you.

Stress also has side benefits. For example, your body will be stronger if you have both times of calm and periods of heart-pounding excitement: Research shows that people with no variability in their heart rate have a higher risk of death from a number of causes. Stress also improves your performance. More than one hundred years ago, psychologists Robert M. Yerkes and J. D. Dodson demonstrated the scientific principle that people work better under stress, which explains the phenomenon of people like Susan, who always got better grades on her term papers when she started writing them the night before they were due.

However, there are limits to the positive effects of stress. The Yerkes-Dodson law proves that once stress reaches a certain point, productivity goes down. Sports coaches have relied on this principle for decades, deliberately stressing their teams with aggressive, bullying pregame talks, but also easing up when necessary. If the players are revved up, they'll play better. But if they are too anxious, they will literally drop the ball. Naturally, people are different in what makes them stressed and how much stress they can tolerate before their productivity declines. This explains the other phenomenon of people like Ali, who always wrote terrible papers if she waited until the night before they were due. There is also a point where stress stops being healthy. In the short term, too much stress can lead to sleep problems and irritability. When stress is severe and prolonged, it is linked to high blood pressure, heart problems, and a weakened immune system.

If you want a Pretty Healthy life, your goal is not to completely avoid stress and lounge in your pj's all day. Not only is the couch-potato life boring, it's a classic sign of clinical depression. Your goal is to bring on a reasonable amount of challenge and excitement— and amass a repertoire of strategies to keep you from being overwhelmed when life throws you too many curveballs.

Quiz: Is Your Stress Level Pretty Healthy?

When you are under a lot of stress, your body sends up red flags. Headaches, backaches, insomnia, and irritability are all signs of stress overload. These stress symptoms can be medi-

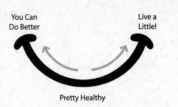

You Can Do Better

Live a Little!

Pretty Healthy

cated out of existence with alcohol, sleeping pills, over-the-counter pain relievers, or antianxiety drugs. Wanting to eliminate your symptoms is understandable—after all, no one wants to feel bad—but beware of masking what's really going on in your life. The quiz below is designed to help you tune in to your body's signals. It will also help you understand when you've crossed the line between stress that keeps you on your toes and stress that trips you up. For each sign of stress, circle the statement that most closely describes how you feel. Then tally up your numbers and read about your score.

Stress Symptoms:

Sleeping Problems

0 points. You have the kind of deep, trouble-free sleep that most people only dream about. Sometimes your friends or family complain that you sleep *too* much.

1 point. Most nights you sleep well, but every now and then your worries keep you awake. You may be tired the next day, but a brisk walk or short jog can get your blood flowing again.

2 points. You often have trouble falling asleep or staying asleep—or both. Maybe you even sleep a lot more than you used to. Either way, you just don't feel like getting out of bed in the morning.

(continued)

3 points. It's really, really hard for you to sleep at night. You spend the days dreading your sleepless nights, and you spend your nights afraid that you will be exhausted during the day to come.

Pain

0 points. What pain? You pride yourself on never taking any medication.

1 point. You have some occasional muscle pain (headache, clenched jaw, backache) that can't be explained by an injury or illness, but in general you feel pretty good.

2 points. Most days find you coping with serious aches and pains, but you can still do the things you enjoy. You tend to feel better on weekends or on days when you have less to do.

3 points. You hurt nearly every day, and sometimes the pain is so debilitating you take to your bed. People may even accuse you of exaggerating your pain to get attention.

Gastrointestinal Distress

0 points. You and your cast-iron stomach can scarf down a meal of spicy chili and wash it down with red wine, with no unpleasant digestive consequences. Hey, was that chocolate cake on the dessert cart?

1 point. Although your GI system is more sensitive than it used to be, things function pretty smoothly most of the time.

2 points. You have so much indigestion that you've started checking the labels on your antacids to be sure you don't exceed the maximum dose.

3 points. You know your GI doctor by his first name. You've swallowed so much barium that you glow in the dark, but despite all your medical workups, there appears to be no organic cause for your distress.

(continued)

Depression

0 points. You don't have all that much to do, and yet every little chore feels like a huge burden.

1 point. You meet your daily challenges with a bounce in your step.

2 points. You can function pretty well, but everything takes a lot more effort than it used to. You rarely feel genuinely happy.

3 points. You feel hopeless about the future; what is there to look forward to? You've stopped doing the things that once brought you joy.

Anxiety

0 points. You're supercool. Your friends joke about how nothing seems to faze you.

1 point. Life feels like a roller-coaster ride. It's sometimes scary, sometimes thrilling, and mostly fun.

2 points. You worry about things—such as the possibility of getting cancer or that your child will fail in school—without good reason. Friends comment on how jumpy you are.

3 points. You are constantly hyperalert and hypervigilant. You can't even imagine what it's like not to feel anxious all the time.

Irritability

0 points. You're nice to everyone, even the phone solicitors who call at dinnertime. Sure, you'd love to participate in a market survey!

1 point. Sometimes you are irritated for no good reason. You snap at someone and later think to yourself, "Wow, I really overreacted. What's up with that?"

2 points. You're crabby more often than you're nice.

(continued)

3 points. You are a bitch on wheels. Yelling at the people you love isn't satisfying enough, so you also yell at sales clerks, kids on scooters, and television characters.

Exercise Habits

0 points. You exercise regularly, and you love every sweaty minute.

1 point. It takes self-discipline, but you stick to an exercise routine and like how good it makes you feel.

2 points. You often find excuses not to exercise. "Life is hard," you tell yourself. "I deserve a break."

3 points. For you, exercise is a matter of extremes. Either you force yourself to run four miles despite a stress fracture and a bad case of the flu—or you give up completely and donate all your workout clothes to Goodwill.

Eating Junk Food

0 points. Junk food is not a temptation for you. At the sandwich shop, you always choose a side of fruit instead of potato chips.

1 point. You relish the occasional Big Mac after a bad day at work, and you know that an indulgence now and then won't kill you.

2 points. You're concerned about how much junk food you're eating, but you look on the bright side: At least you still have the self-control to top your ice cream with bananas instead of Cool Whip.

3 points. Again, extremes rule the day. Either junk food is both your escape and your best friend—*or* you are so obsessed with a "pure" diet that you agonize for weeks if a gram of trans fat passes your lips.

Loss of Libido

0 points. Sex? You can take it or leave it. Whatever.

1 point. You don't seem to have sex as often as you used to, but you're happy with your new philosophy of "quality over quantity."

(continued)

2 points. You can still be persuaded to have sex, but you don't take as much pleasure in it as you used to. Achieving orgasm is difficult, if not impossible.

3 points. The thought of someone touching your body makes you want to run screaming from the room.

Lack of Time

0 points. You have more time than you need. Some days, you're bored.

1 point. Your schedule is usually flexible enough to accommodate the activities that nourish your spirit.

2 points. It takes some frantic multitasking, but you can usually meet all of your obligations. You wish you had a few more minutes to unwind at the end of the day.

3 points. You dash from task to task; the things you used to enjoy are now just another set of chores you can't finish. You've canceled dates with your friends so many times, they don't even bother calling you anymore.

Scoring

0–8 points: You are mellow yellow. In fact, you're so relaxed that we have to ask: Are you sure you're getting *enough* stress? Seek out avenues of professional or creative stimulation, even if you have to risk losing some of your legendary cool. If the thought of engaging in activity is repulsive to you, consider that you may be depressed—and check in with a doctor.

9–17 points: You're stressed … *and* you're in the PH Zone. A few headaches or restless nights aren't such a high price to pay for a fulfilling life. If your stress symptoms really bother you, or if they tend to collect all in one area of your life, such as sleep, try some of the stress management techniques in this chapter to help you enjoy the fruits of your hard labor.

(continued)

18–24 points: You're under a high level of stress, and the strain is starting to show. You're still in the PH Zone, but whether you can stay there depends on how long this intense stress will last. If your stress is caused by a temporary situation (your sister just had open-heart surgery, or you're moving to a new house), you'll probably be just fine. Your body is designed to handle a certain amount of psychological strain. But why not learn some stress management techniques? You'll feel a lot better while you get through this period.

If your stress doesn't appear to have an end in sight, you must find ways to reduce your stress and bring more enjoyment into your life. And take heart: A stressful life is not necessarily a ticket to poor health, as long as you find ways to meet your needs. This chapter contains several suggestions for making this happen.

25–30 points: Whoa! It's not easy to impress us with stress levels (we are both intimately acquainted with serious stress), but your score is practically off the charts. Listen up: Your body and mind are telling you that there is far too much stress in your life. It's time to make a dramatic change. Start by adopting the stress management techniques described in this chapter. If those aren't enough, get outside help from a therapist, doctor, or trusted friend to figure out how to increase your coping skills. Consider seeing your primary care physician to evaluate the effects of chronic, sky-high stress on your body.

Stress, Redefined

Most of us think of stress in vague terms: It's something that causes tension and pressure, right? Or it's what happens when there's too much to do. We'd like to propose a tidy definition that pinpoints both a cause and solution: *Stress is the fear that you don't have the resources to successfully meet your challenges.*

What the Health?

When we are first confronted with stress, our immune system is enhanced. But the effect is short-lived, according to Robert Sapolsky's book *Why Zebras Don't Get Ulcers*. After an hour, stress begins to have the opposite effect and suppresses immunity. If you develop serious, long-term stress, the immune system can plummet between 40 and 70 percent below normal.

Interesting, isn't it? According to this definition, stress is not caused by the challenges themselves. It's caused by a perceived shortage of resources—not enough time, not enough money, not enough talent, not enough emotional support. For example, the two of us take on a lot of work each year: writing books, giving talks, traveling . . . in addition to our jobs, homes, and families. It's a good life, but it comes with the fear that we won't have time to get everything done, or that we will have to make unacceptable personal sacrifices to meet our obligations. That's a major source of stress for us. Note that the stress is not caused by our workload itself but by our reactions to it. ("How will I get it all done?" or "What if my plane is late and I have to miss my daughter's school dance?")

This concept applies to life's major challenges as well. When Susan was young, her mother, who was living in Mexico City, had an operation to remove a benign brain tumor. Later, when Susan was fresh out of medical school and chief resident of surgery, a scan showed that the tumor had returned and that her mother would need a second operation. As a newly minted doctor and dutiful daughter, Susan arranged for her mother to fly up to the

States, where better scanning equipment and surgical teams were available—but her mother declined. Instead, Susan and her siblings flew down to Mexico City for the operation. The surgery revealed that the CAT scan was wrong: The tumor had not come back and the operation had been unnecessary. As Susan sat with her mother in the recovery room, her mom complained of a headache. Then she went into cardiac arrest. Susan called for assistance, but her mother fell into a coma. Ten days later, she died. She was fifty-eight years old.

What a tragic situation—and stressful as well, for many reasons, including the emotional free fall of losing a mother. Susan also worried that as the eldest child and as a doctor, she would be expected to step up and act as a guiding presence for her father and four siblings. But Susan didn't feel up to the part, mainly because she blamed herself for not being able to save her mother. If, after all her years of training, she was unable to prevent her mother's death, how would she be able to take care of her family? She felt incompetent and alone. Susan's reality was bad, but her reaction to the reality was worse. She struggled for a long time before she could start forgiving herself for a tragedy that wasn't her responsibility in the first place. Over the years, Susan has grown better at recognizing when she can control events and when she can't. This is an essential skill that doctors develop with time. The rest of us need to learn it as well.

The point of Susan's story is that even in a tragedy, how we cope is determined by our perception of the event. This is not to say that you could avoid stress by having perfect reactions. No one can do that, and no one would *want* to react to a parent's death in a way that didn't produce stress. The point is that if you want to reduce some of your stress, and if stress is caused by your perception that you lack sufficient resources to handle your challenges, then you have a few options on the table.

"No"

Unless you live in an isolation tank, you can't eliminate challenges. But a legitimate way to reduce stress is to reduce the burden you carry, especially if your stress is caused by having too much to do. Lately, we have both worked on ways to cut back on unrewarding activities. Susan maintains a list of her goals for the upcoming year or two, and if an opportunity comes up that doesn't help serve those overarching goals, she simply won't take it.

Life doesn't always present such clear choices, however. Sometimes you have to use other standards to separate the wheat from the chaff on your to-do list. Ali's fall schedule is always both exciting and busy, with conferences or talks on (of all things) stress management nearly every week. When a group of young breast cancer survivors asked if she would donate her time one September to give a talk on self-nurturance, Ali agreed to the request. Presenting the talk meant that Ali would have to give up another night with her young children, but the cause was a good one. Ali made room in her schedule and gave the talk—only to find herself heckled by a woman in her seventies, who was irate that Ali's lecture hadn't addressed the needs of elderly women. Somehow it had escaped the heckler that the audience was supposed to be made up entirely of *young* survivors. Comedians may be practiced at handling disruptive audience members, but to Ali, who was giving the talk as a free service, this was both out of the blue and really unpleasant. To make matters worse, no one from the group's organizing committee stopped the woman or offered an apology to Ali afterward. Instead of feeling useful and uplifted, Ali went home feeling tired, unappreciated, and sad that she had missed time with her kids.

Afterward, Ali's husband said, "Why did you put yourself through this? You didn't get paid—you didn't even get a pot of flowers—and now you're exhausted *and* you've been angered by a woman who wasn't even supposed to be there in the first place." He was right, and this event drove home the point he'd been making for years: that the advantages of a busy lecture season are not always greater than the disadvantages. Now Ali very carefully weighs the full repercussions of saying yes to a request, even if it's for a good cause. Which brings us to the delicate matter of saying no.

Everyone knows that stress reduction sometimes means saying no—to the requests to bill more hours, organize the Memorial Day fun run, host the day-after-Thanksgiving breakfast for the extended family. Yet the word "no" doesn't slip easily past most women's lips, mainly because no one ever taught us how to say it well.

Take some time now to learn this life skill. Imagine that someone has asked you to make brownies for the bake sale tomorrow. You

What the Health?

Denial isn't always unhealthy. In fact, just the opposite. Sometimes it's also a girl's best friend. In a 1999 study published in *Cancer Investigation,* cancer patients who used denial as a coping technique were much less anxious than those who employed problem-solving methods to handle their tension.

don't want to do it. Here are some of our favorite ways for getting past even the most persistent bake sale hostess:

- **Just say no.** Responding to requests with a list of timid excuses and hesitant apologies doesn't work. Usually, the person making the request will smell your fear and press you even harder. It is both refreshing and effective to say nothing but no, and leave it at that.

- **No, sorry, can't do it right now.** This is a version of "Just say no," toned down with an apology, albeit a brisk one.

- **No, because . . .** As in, "No, because I'm sick" or "No, because I have a presentation to give at work tomorrow and don't have time to bake." Be prepared for the possibility that the bake sale hostess will swoop in with a "solution" to your excuse. ("You're sick? That's okay; you can use these food service gloves and no one will get your germs!") But often people appreciate a short, simple reason for a turndown.

- **No, but how about . . . ?** Here, you offer a substitute that you can live with. "No, but how about I help out at next month's fundraiser?" or "No, but how about I pick up some paper plates and napkins for you at the store instead?" This works only if you really, truly want to do what you suggest.

- **I don't have my appointment book with me. Can you e-mail me?** By putting space between the request and your answer, you reduce the chances that you will sputter "Yes!" out of sheer panic. Plus, it's much easier to decline by return e-mail than in person.

- **Let me check with my assistant/boss/partner/kids first.** When you involve another person, you shift some of the burden away from yourself. Susan likes this strategy because she doesn't keep her own schedule (so she really does have to check with her assistant) and because the choices she makes have repercussions for her entire family. Play fair here, and don't use someone else as a cover for a lie.

• **No, because I have a policy about . . .** A rejection is less personal if you apply it to everyone. "No, because I don't bake," or "No, because I don't donate my time on weekdays, just weekends."

Expand Your Resources

A few years ago, Ali was driving through New Hampshire with her husband, Dave. It was October and the leaves were brilliant shades of orange, red, and yellow . . . but Ali's mood was black. Dave quickly became aware of said mood and, praying that it was caused by PMS and not something he had done, chose his words carefully for most of the trip. But then he said something terrible.

"Isn't the view gorgeous?" he asked.

Ali snarled back with what was, clearly, the only logical response: "You are just not meeting my needs!"

Dave, feeling brave, took a deep breath and said, "Okay. What are those needs?"

Ali turned to him. *"I don't know!"* she wailed.

The lesson of this story? There are three.

Lesson number one: *No one can meet your needs until you know what they are.* If stress is caused by your fear that you don't have enough resources to meet your challenges, stress reduction starts with understanding what it is you lack. So go ahead and write down whatever it is you need. Go ahead and define "need" loosely to include not just the things you absolutely require for bare-bones survival but also whatever would make your particular challenges a lot easier to face. These needs can be physical, emotional, financial . . . whatever. If you have school-age children and the thought of getting through the homework/dinner/bath/bedtime crush makes your right shoulder blade start to twitch, consider what you need to make it through the evening. Do you need more help getting dinner on the table? Someone to massage your back? Or just a little recognition for your daily heroism?

Once you know what you-need, you're in a much better position to figure out how to get that need taken care of. Remember, stress is caused by a *perceived* lack of resources. When you make your list, it will hopefully become apparent that you are surrounded by resources, perhaps even swimming in resources—in the form of family, friends, and colleagues. Yes, it's perfectly okay to ask other people to help you meet your challenges. But be careful, because here comes the next lesson:

Lesson number two: *You can't expect one person to meet all your needs.* Ali not only wanted Dave to telepathically sense all her needs—even the ones she couldn't identify—she also expected him to satisfy each and every one of them. Without realizing it, Ali was buying in to one of the most damaging myths of our times, the one that says your life partner should grant you ultimate fulfillment. That's right: The famous line "You complete me" is, sadly, wishful thinking.

If you don't believe us, think back a generation or two. Your mother or grandmother may have been stifled by her lack of choices and quite probably yearned for greater intellectual or creative stimulation. But she probably also enjoyed a sense of community that is harder for us to achieve today. Even though the two of us grew up in very different places (Ali in Massachusetts, Susan in Mexico), our mothers each were part of a circle of neighborhood women who met for coffee while we and our friends played in another room. They also had volunteer work that drew them together with other women in similar situations. While working for the school, hospital, church, or synagogue, they could talk with women who had some of the same joys and problems they had. In even earlier generations, women could kvetch while making quilts or canning vegetables. They spent enough time together that they could make an educated guess about who needed a little extra help with the kids or the sewing, and who needed a good cry.

Few of us want to return to prefeminist days, and canning vegetables in a hot kitchen is a pretty sweaty job even when you have friends around, but let's be honest: Even as women have grown less dependent on men financially, we have become more dependent emotionally. Without the time to nurture our friendships, we've come to expect significant others to be not just lovers and helpmates but best friends, career counselors, and spiritual guides. That's an unfair burden to place on any single person. It strains relationships and sets us up for the stress created by unmet needs.

The problem is not men and their supposed emotional shortcomings. We often hear women say, "Oh, if my husband were only a woman, he'd understand everything about me." That's just not true. If you talk to women in lesbian relationships, you'll learn that they have the very same problem of wondering why the other person doesn't "get" them. The same can happen outside of romantic relationships, when in friendships we mistakenly think that a true friend should supply us with all the missing pieces of our life's puzzle.

So look at your list of needs, and, if you're in a romantic relationship, think carefully about which of them your partner can realistically meet. Maybe your husband is never going to be a great cheerleader for you, or maybe he gets home from work too late to make dinner. So . . . don't expect those things from him. But he might be delighted to rub out the kinks in your shoulder at the end of the night. For the other items, look around. You'll probably find plenty of friends or family members who will be happy to help you meet your other needs. People love to do what they're good at, so call your excitable friend when you need someone to be happy for you. Ask your mother to make an extra batch of her chicken noodle soup that you can pull out of the freezer on desperate nights.

Of course, sometimes the reason you're stressed is because you don't have a supportive family or many friends. Maybe you've just moved to a new town, or you're shy, or your friends just aren't emotionally available. Most of Susan's friends are men she knows from work. They're great for professional camaraderie and joking around, but they're not big on cozy, sympathetic talks over tea. For Susan, her church and the people in it have turned out to be an important resource. If you were raised in a religious tradition and haven't revisited it for a while, consider going back. Churches, synagogues, and mosques have changed since you were a kid, and so have you. Some of what you objected to in your teens or twenties might be gone now, and in their place you may discover a source of great comfort and community. You can also follow the principle that like appeals to like. In other words, you may find friends just by doing what you like to do, whether it's running, folk dancing, or bird-watching. If you can't get out of the house easily, you can find many communities online. Chatting online may not be the same as having someone to hold your hand, but perhaps it's better than being alone.

Lesson number three: *Ask for what you need.* We joke about men who won't ask for directions, but women have a bigger hang-up: We won't ask for help. We feel guilty and ashamed, even morally weak, about not being able to do everything alone. If you want to reduce your stress, you have to change this way of thinking. You can start by recognizing some basic facts about human nature. Most of us enjoy helping others, and there's nothing we hate more than watching helplessly from the sidelines as our loved ones suffer. When you ask for help, you're giving your friends or family the gift of being needed.

You can also take turns giving and receiving. Ali, who has a new puppy, just asked a neighbor who works from home if she can take the dog out this Friday. In return, she will bake the neighbor a loaf of banana bread. In other cases, it can be years or decades between turns, but the result is even more profound. When Susan's mother died, an aunt paid for Susan's sister to go to college. Now Susan repays the favor by footing the tuition bill for another young relative. She hopes that in the future, the next generation will help out one of their young nieces or nephews in a similar way. Accepting help, and agreeing to pay back the debt that goes with it, is a way of living generously.

When you are in a real crisis, knowing how to ask for help can make the difference between staying afloat and sinking. This is true even when you are surrounded by people who are eager to help you, as they don't always know what you need and are left to figure it out on their own. This is the "casserole syndrome" that Susan sees in women who are newly diagnosed with breast cancer. Their friends want to help, but they don't know what to do . . . and that's how the woman ends up with thirty casseroles in her freezer, instead of what she really needs, which is someone to pick up her kids from school while she visits the doctor.

In times of serious trouble, it's even more important to figure out what you need and make that list. If someone asks, "What can I do?" look down your list for something that matches up with the person's

abilities. Or, if you've got a close cir[...]
other, give the list to one friend who [...]
else. They can divide up the items as t[...]
calculating to you, consider how help[...]
need but you don't know what to do. V[...]
a list of the things that would make a d[...]

with) and some[...]
two in the[...]
doesn't[...]
you[...]

Happy or Cr[...]

We want you to be happy . . . within limits. Most of us have a baseline mood that is neither blissful nor morose. It's a state that allows for everyday ups, downs, disappointments, fears, and joys, but mostly it's neutral. This baseline state is Pretty Healthy! Drug companies have led us to expect superhappiness on a daily basis, but that's not normal. That's manic. So instead of careening from one source of excitement to another in the hopes of a happiness buzz, focus on achieving your real goals. Then you will know the more profound states of contentment and peace of mind.

Finally—although this is by no means a last resort—you can also pay for help. Buying a takeout dinner can be a sign that you're a good strategist, not that you are a failure as a mother and a chef. Paying a massage therapist to work on your sore muscles may be more efficient than spending hours cajoling a reluctant partner into rubbing your shoulders.

Resources You Carry with You

We are both blessed to have wonderful families and plenty of friends. Some of these friends are party friends (who are really fun to be

...are foxhole friends (the ones you can call in tears at ...morning). Some are both. But there are times when it ...matter how many or what kind of friends you have, because ...are saddled with a problem that no one else can make better. During these times, you need to draw on your internal resources.

Your internal resources include personality traits, such as intelligence, persistence, courage, and toughness; skills you possess; and the wisdom you've accumulated over the years. When you start to feel stressed, take a good hard look at the challenges you face and ask if you really, truly believe that you lack the internal resources to cope with them. As an example, let's take a classically stressful situation: You're in the grocery store with a two-year-old who is throwing a temper tantrum. As the child screams, your heart starts to pound and you feel your blood pressure rise. This is a good time to ask whether you have the resources to cope with the challenge:

Do you have the courage to ignore the other shoppers' judgments about your child and your parenting skills? Check.

Do you have experience defusing explosive situations? Check.

Do you have enough patience to push the cart and your child through four more aisles without completely losing it? Hmmm. Let's try another one.

Do you know a few stress management techniques, such as deep breathing, that can patch up your worn-out patience? Ah, yes. Check. (For some specific stress management techniques, keep reading.)

By matching your internal resources to the challenges at hand, you give stress a lot less power to undermine you. If you don't know your own strengths, though, they can't help you. This is probably one of the reasons both men and women grow so much happier with age. Their life experiences have shown them they can handle a variety of challenges, so there's less need to sweat the small stuff, and even the big stuff becomes less frightening.

Even if you lack certain useful traits, such as a cool temperament or the ability to program your cell phone's address book, you can always cultivate new ones. More important, you can certainly learn a handful of techniques to expand your collection of stress management skills. The techniques that follow can help you feel calmer and more peaceful almost immediately, but even better is their carryover effect. If you perform one of these techniques three or four times a week, you will soon become less reactive to stress in general.

Here are some of our favorite stress management techniques:

Meditation. Meditation is famous for eliciting the relaxation response, a state in which your body becomes less sensitive to adrenaline and less jumpy. Yet people get very stressed out at the thought of meditation because it seems to require so much discipline. It's not hard. Really. Start by finding a quiet place to sit where you won't be interrupted. Think of a mantra, which is a sound, word, or phrase that has a peaceful or neutral meaning to you. The classic mantra is the sound "ohm," but you can also try "stillness" or "calm blue ocean," or anything that feels right. Mindfully take a breath and say your mantra to yourself; exhale and say it again. Repeat this for fifteen to twenty minutes, trying to keep your focus on your mantra. You will almost certainly discover that your attention wanders. That's okay; every time this happens, gently bring your attention back to your mantra. Although no one has perfect focus, you will grow more and more comfortable with meditation as you continue its practice.

Guided imagery. Imagine yourself in a calming situation, perhaps relaxing in a field of wildflowers or standing at the edge of a beach. Use each of your senses to put yourself fully into the scene. Can you smell the mild perfume of the flowers? Is the water warm as it laps against your toes? Spend as much time as you like in this scene. Know that you can return to this peaceful place at any time, even if it's just for a moment or two between meetings.

Progressive muscle relaxation (PMR). Described on pages 44–45, PMR is especially effective at improving sleep and reducing muscle tension.

Focused breathing. You know that deep, abdominal breathing is good for you, but in a time of crisis it's only natural to gulp down air in shallow, unsatisfying breaths. So when you are stressed, gently turn your focus to your breathing. Slow it down by mentally counting "one, two, three, four" while you inhale. When you exhale, count "four, three, two, one." Breathe deeply from your diaphragm. If this is hard for you, try heaving a big sigh. *Voilà!* You just breathed from your diaphragm.

Keeping a journal. Expressing your emotions in writing can be highly beneficial to your health. In a study published in the journal *Stress, Immunity, and Health,* students were asked to write in a journal for four successive days for twenty minutes at a time. They were assigned to write about either traumatic events in their lives or emotionally neutral ones. Six months later, the students who had written about traumatic events were happier and less depressed than the students in the neutral group. They had better immune function as well. Ali asks most of her patients to keep a journal when they're having a tough time, and they report the results are cathartic. "The journal helps me let my worries go," some women have said to Ali; others say, "It brings me insight."

Exercise. Stop thinking of exercise as a way to punish yourself for eating (or as an excuse for eating more) and start thinking of it as a stress management technique. Although it's a more vigorous way to reduce stress than the other techniques listed here, exercise has the same ability to make you feel better almost instantly. That effect generalizes itself to your entire week when you exercise regularly. There are several studies about the great reasons to exercise, but we really like one that was performed at Duke University in 2007 that shows exercise to be just as effective as medication in reducing depression, which is a common consequence of severe stress.

To really work out your stress, try an exercise that requires serious cardiovascular effort, such as power walking up and down a hilly neighborhood, dancing, swimming, or cycling. You can also try an activity like power yoga, which combines the focus of meditation with the intensity of a cardiovascular workout.

Susan's Story: If I'm Stressed, It Must Be October

In October, which is breast cancer awareness month, I am very busy with speaking engagements, media appearances, and other events. I don't have time to exercise or meditate or do the other nonwork things I enjoy. My life starts to feel like that drawer in the kitchen where you stuff everything you don't know what to do with. You shove more and more stuff into the drawer . . . and then one day you open the drawer and everything falls out onto the floor.

When that happens, I have to accept that I might not have time to organize the drawer that very day. I probably won't have time to deal with the drawer until October is over. You probably have your own version of October, whether it's the holidays or the end of the fiscal year or whatever. If you want to pull through times of massive but temporary stress, you need to remember that there's a light at the end of the tunnel. What I do in October is think about how I will organize my life in November, when things are calmer.

That's why I love to make lists. When I'm sitting on a plane in October, flying toward a meeting or lecture and feeling my stress rising, I pull out my notebook and make lists of things I need to do. Acute items go in the front of the notebook; long-term goals are in the back. Just having everything written down makes me feel much better, even though I won't get around to most of the items for weeks, if not months. And sometimes making lists helps me see that certain items just aren't worth worrying about, because I realize that they will take less time than I thought, or because there's no way I can get to them anytime in the next year.

I'm also famous for my color-coded schedules, which are really fantasies in which I decide in the best of all worlds how my days will unfold. In my ideal life, I get up at six to exercise and medi-tate; then I respond to e-mails from the East Coast; at nine o'clock I start my conference calls; and so on. Even after October is fin-ished, these schedules rarely work out exactly the way I want them to, but that's not the point. I don't force myself or other people to adhere to them. They're for my comfort in the middle of a stressful time, and they reassure me that I will eventually find time for the things I like to do.

Not everyone likes schedules. Some people are stressed out by schedules because once something is on paper they feel they have to stick with it. And some people just don't find lists as soothing as I do. Whenever my daughter complains about being overwhelmed, I say, "Make a list!" And she looks at me like I'm crazy. It doesn't work for her. But it might work for her later in life, because as you get older a source of stress is that you're afraid of forgetting what you're supposed to do. When your tasks are written down you don't have to worry about that anymore!

Perfectionism Alert: The PBW

We want you to aim for a good level of stress in your life. But we don't want this goal to become a source of stress in itself. We can't help but notice that although relaxation ought to be, um, relaxing, stress management has somehow become yet another pressing item on a woman's to-do list. It's as if the 1990s image of the Superwoman who could effortlessly juggle family and career has been replaced by the Perfectly Balanced Woman. The PBW is never psychotically busy but is also never bored; she always makes time for the yoga classes that refresh her soul and lend a rosy glow to her skin. She never scowls at her coworkers; she doesn't need to stagger into Starbucks in the late afternoon, desperate for a hit of caffeine and sugar. And she never inconveniences her family by taking to bed with a tension headache. Did we mention that she can wear

Stress Myths versus Stress Realities

Myth: Stress causes cancer.

Reality: A lot of women who get cancer feel guilty because someone has told them that cancer is the result of their "toxic thoughts"
or their inability to manage stress. This is a shame, because no one
needs to feel guilty about getting cancer.

The truth is more nuanced. There is evidence that many or most
of us are walking around today with dormant cancer cells in our bodies. And we're absolutely fine . . . unless something happens to wake
those cells up. One theory is that changes in the body's environment
can trigger the awakening of these cells. What kind of changes? Well,
we know that within a year after the death of a spouse, the surviv-
ing partner has an increased risk of death from cancer and other
problems. So it's possible that extreme, long-term stress can create
the conditions that allow cancer cells to flourish. Keep in mind that
this is only a theory. There's no reason to believe that more moderate
amounts of stress lead to cancer.

Myth: Stress can give you a heart attack.

Reality: Actually, this isn't a myth. Long-term stress can lead to
high blood pressure and cardiovascular problems such as angina.
And if your heart isn't so good in the first place, both extreme anger
and extreme joy can place too much demand on a weakened ticker
and actually precipitate sudden cardiac death. Those of us who are
basically healthy do not have to worry about intense but brief encounters with extreme emotions. Also, keep in mind that the temporary stress of a few crazy-busy weeks are unlikely to have negative
long-term effects on your heart.

Myth: Exercise is always the best way to reduce stress.

Reality: The stress-relieving effects of exercise have been well
documented, but those effects appear to be reversed if you feel com-

(continued)

pelled to work out against your will. In a famous study performed at the University of Colorado at Boulder, lab rats who were allowed to voluntarily run on a wheel at times of their choosing showed increased measures of health. Rats who were forced to run, however, experienced more sickness. For those of us who don't live in a Habitrail, here's how to apply these findings: Although it's okay to push yourself to work out on days when you feel a little tired or cranky, problems may arise when on a consistent basis your only reason for working out is to please someone else—like angrily dragging yourself to the gym after your partner says you look fat.

Myth: The only way to reduce stress is to tackle your problems head-on.

Reality: If you can address the root cause of your stress, that's great. But sometimes life hands you problems you simply can't fix, such as the serious illness of a loved one. At these times, the best you can do is to manage your response to the situation—which, in fact, can greatly reduce your stress.

adorable stretchy workout pants to her yoga classes because she never, ever needs to indulge in stress eating? The PBW would certainly never eat an entire Pepperidge Farm coconut layer cake straight out of the freezer. Not that we would know anything about what it's like to eat a whole coconut layer cake. (We prefer chocolate.)

If you ever meet a PBW, let us know. We'll let *her* write the stress management chapter for the next edition of this book. However, we're pretty sure that the PBW, like the Superwoman of the 1990s and the Happy Homemaker of the 1950s, is just another myth. She simply doesn't exist. Nevertheless, she makes us feel like failures if we can't live in a constant state of blissful balance. It's no longer enough to suffer from stress-related tension headaches—now we get to feel guilty for having the headaches in the first place.

Know this: Sometimes stress will get the better of you. It happens to both of us all the time. We've already talked about how Ali, despite having devoted her career to stress management, sometimes yells at the people she loves. For her part, Susan has an unfortunate tendency to rear-end the cars in front of her when she's under pressure. A crucial aspect of stress management is self-acceptance—knowing that you are, perhaps, a stress eater. So there may be days when you are so tense and frustrated that you eat a pound of fettuccine Alfredo. It happens. Do what you can to prevent these reactions to stress in the future—meditate, keep a food diary—and then move on. And if you find yourself driving through Los Angeles in the month of October, watch your back.

Chapter Four

Health Screenings:
Do You Really Need a
Baseline Mammogram?

MOST OF US WANT TO take a rational, informed approach to self-care, and what seems more rational and informed than getting regular checkups, mammograms, and other health screenings? At their best, these tests save lives by giving us a heads-up about a disease so that we can deal with it swiftly. But we also have to be fully informed about what is often called "preventive" care.

First, it's not necessarily preventive. Most health screenings detect conditions that already exist; they don't keep those conditions from developing. It's easy to blur this distinction, unconsciously believing something along the lines of "If I get a mammogram every year, I won't get breast cancer." This illusion of control can be dangerous, because if you *are* diagnosed with a problem, you can wrongly feel you're to blame. ("If only I hadn't postponed my screening by two months!") Losing this false sense of control can be such a devastating shock that it can blunt your ability to marshal your resources and cope with the diagnosis.

Obscuring the distinction between prevention and detection can also distract you from doing things that truly are preventive. These include the mundane but absolutely crucial precautions of wearing a seat belt, practicing safe sex, and not smoking. These habits are the best ways to prevent disability or a premature death. So get your mammograms—in this chapter, we'll talk about reasonable schedules for these and other screenings—but don't forget to wear your seat belt on the way there.

Screenings Should Lead to Better Outcomes

To make things more complicated, it's usually good for a patient when a health screening detects an asymptomatic condition—but not always. Examples of the positive power of early detection include a reduced risk of stroke in people who lower their high blood pressure or, in the case of colon and cervical cancers, the treatment of potentially cancerous growths via minor surgery. Isn't it amazing that we can undergo a health screening that reveals a possibly cancerous lesion, have it removed under local anesthetic, and come home to our own snug beds—sometimes all in the same day?

But being thankful doesn't mean we also have to be blind to the fact that some asymptomatic conditions never turn into problems at all. There are times when it is much better not to know about these conditions in the first place. A randomized, controlled study in

Japan found that neuroblastoma, a solid cancer that appears in early childhood, can be detected by testing acid levels in the urine of infants. Because neuroblastoma can be treated in its very early stages, but is almost always fatal later on, the Japanese government instituted a massive screening program in which parents sent in samples of their babies' urine for testing. As was expected, many more tumors were discovered in their early stages. What was unexpected was that mortality rates from neuroblastoma did not go down. They stayed about the same. The study's researchers concluded that the program unearthed many tumors that did not turn out to be clinically relevant, meaning that they would have never developed into cancer. This mighty screening effort did not lead to longer lives for more children. It just led to more babies having operations they didn't need. Because surgery has inherent risks, including infection and complications from anesthesia, this is a case of screening that could have easily done more harm than good.

Whole-body CAT scans delivered a similar lesson. Although whole-body CAT scans deliver a wallop of radiation (its doses are far higher than what you get during a chest X-ray or mammogram), they were all the rage several years ago. In major cities, you could find scanning boutiques open for business on street corners. The promise was that you could be fully scanned for previously undetected maladies and get treated quickly—or, alternatively, you'd get a completely reassuring bill of health. What usually happened, however, was in the unpleasant middle. Physical quirks tended to show up on the scans, and, inevitably, these quirks required further screenings and surgeries to rule out possible problems. Many patients found the follow-up process so long, grueling, and ultimately such a waste of time and money that the scans have fallen out of favor.

So we can't assume that more screenings are always better, or that finding more tumors, lesions, or growths will prevent more deaths. We have to subject our tests and procedures to review, asking not just whether they detect potential problems but whether they lead to better outcomes for the people who get them. We also have to take into account the risk and stress posed by the screenings and the treatments that may follow.

Do I Really Need to Get a Physical Every Year?

The annual physical used to be a cornerstone of "preventive" medicine, but today you'll hear a variety of opinions about how often to see your doctor for a checkup. We asked the BeWell Experts to hash out the question: Is an annual physical really necessary?

NANCY SNYDERMAN: It depends on how you define "physical." I think you should check in with your doctor annually. There are things about us that change from year to year, both physically and socially. It doesn't mean that we need the kind of full-body checkups that doctors were taught to do in the fifties. Maybe it means getting your blood pressure checked or having a urinalysis. But there should be an annual connection with someone.

SUSAN: But there's no data that physicals change health outcomes at all.

ALI: I also think you should check in with your physician at least once a year. At the least, you should get your blood pressure checked. I see my doctor at least once a year, because, as Nancy said, things do change.

NANCY SNYDERMAN: Things change that you don't see, but your doctor might.

ALI: And what if you've been on a medication for ten years and it turns out there is something else now that's better or less expensive?

SUSAN: I think you put too much faith in your doctor!

LORETTA LAROCHE: A checkup should be about more than just your physical well-being. I wish doctors would ask their patients if they felt supported and loved. They should ask if their patients are engaged in something they feel passionate about, if they laugh often, if they feel that life has purpose. If the answers are no, life can feel "life less."

ALI: For a while I went in only when I was sick, but when you're there for a specific problem the doctor just whips in, checks your symptoms, and whips out. Whatever you're complaining about is all the doctor focuses on.

LORETTA LAROCHE: I grew up in a family that didn't go to the doctor unless they were almost dead, and my mom is ninety-seven.

SUSAN: Exactly. I think doctors can be bad for you. And a risk is that you'll go and have a routine test that labels you with a disease like osteopenia, which is not a disease at all—it just means that you have a slight loss of bone mass, and doesn't necessarily increase your chances of having a fracture—and then you're on the merry road toward treating a problem that wasn't really a problem in the first place.

CHRIS ECONOMOS: I think you should check in with *someone*. I've been seeing a doctor regularly for a while, and the questions she asks always lead to something positive.

HOPE RICCIOTTI: I'm with Susan on this one. We don't have evidence that physicals are going to keep all of us healthy. It depends on what *you* need. Young women need annual Paps, people with hypertension need to get their blood pressure checked more often, and so on. But we have only a certain number of dollars to spend on health care, and the dollars we do spend ought to be based on the evidence.

NANCY SNYDERMAN: We have to change our concept of the annual physical. I'm not suggesting that we all need traditional physicals with a doctor who checks your ears, throat, skin, and everything else. I'm thinking of a visit that's tailored to the patient's needs. If you're at risk for melanoma, then maybe you want someone to check your skin every year.

SUSAN: Especially if you live alone and don't have someone who looks at your back now and then.

MIM NELSON: But when we talk about the value of physicals, I think of my father. He smoked and drank, even though his dad died of a heart attack. When he was forty-eight, my dad went in for an annual physical and the doctor said, "You have a choice. You can be dead within three years, or you can clean up your act." Now my dad is getting ready to turn eighty! I'm thankful there was a physician who gave him the opportunity to change.

SUSAN: But to make every single person have an annual physical just because a small percentage will benefit . . . that doesn't seem right.

MIM NELSON: The women who will read this book are smart. They can figure out how to use the health care system.

SUSAN: Yes!

False Positives

Another factor to consider when you are evaluating whether to undergo a health screening is the number of false positives it tends to produce. False positives, which are results that erroneously suggest

you have a disease, can lead to worrisome, expensive workups or surgeries whose main purpose is to prove that nothing bad is going on.

Breast self-exams are a good example of how a screening technique can become entrenched in our medical system even if it produces more false positives than an equally effective alternative. The
formal breast self-exam was born in the 1950s, because doctors
were concerned about the number of women who delayed treatment until their cancers were at a very late stage, with tumors that
were large and ulcerating. The doctors concluded that women were
not touching their breasts. If they had, the doctors believed, the
women would have discovered the lumps when they were smaller
and come in earlier, right?

Looking back, the two of us aren't so sure that women really
failed to notice cancers growing in their breasts. In the 1950s, the
only treatment available for a lump was radical mastectomy, and
even then the patient often died. Honestly, if you found a lump
under these conditions, would *you* rush in to see your M.D.? It's our
guess that women were perfectly aware that lumps were forming
in their breasts and growing larger, but the options were so terrible
that they put off seeing a doctor.

Whatever the case may be, breast surgeons of the era responded
by designing the formal breast self-exam (BSE). Over the decades,
women were encouraged to perform BSEs every month as a way
to "prevent" breast cancer, and by the 1990s a minor industry had
grown up around BSEs, selling special pads to make the BSE more
comfortable or shower cards that showed how to perform BSEs—
exactly where to touch your breasts, in what sequence you should
touch each area, how to move your fingers, and so on. It was rarely
mentioned that there was no evidence to back up the usefulness of
these exams.

Then in 2002 came the results of a very large, well-controlled study of BSEs in China, where the funds for routine mammography aren't available. One group of women was given detailed instruction in BSE and even had to pass a videotaped test to prove their proficiency. These women were also given refresher courses every two years. A second group of women served as a control. Instead of learning to examine their breasts, they were given classes on the unrelated subject of proper techniques for lifting heavy items. Neither group received routine mammograms. At the end of ten years, the BSE group had found more growths—but both groups of women experienced the same number of cancers, at the same stages, and with the same survival rate. The only difference between the two groups was that the BSE women had almost twice as many unnecessary breast biopsies as a result of false positives.

So the BSE turned out not to be so great at reducing breast cancer deaths, but it is really terrific at giving us unnecessary procedures and a lot more stress. The women in the control group found their own cancers, just not doing formal breast self-exams. Now we know that formal BSEs aren't necessary; the ordinary, common poking around we all do is just as good at finding lumps that have clinical relevance.

When More Is Not Better

The "more is not always better" philosophy applies to what is currently our best tool against breast cancer: mammograms. In women over age fifty, mammograms repeatedly have been shown to cut the death rate from breast cancer by 30 percent. In this population, mammograms every year or two make good sense, even though we should all be aware that false positives are part and parcel of mammography, as they occur about 10 percent of the time.

In younger women, the story is a little different. To begin with, their overall risk from breast cancer is lower. The often-cited statistic that one in eight women will develop breast cancer doesn't do a good job of conveying reality. The risk of breast cancer varies a great deal with age, and younger women are not at extraordinarily high levels of risk. According to data from the American Cancer Society, a forty-year-old woman has a 1 in 69 chance of developing breast cancer over the next ten years. At age thirty, her chances are only 1 in 251.

Young women also have denser breast tissue, which means that any tumors that do exist are very hard to see on a mammography screen. In women under forty, looking for tumors in a mammogram is like trying to find polar bears in the snow. Some doctors advise having a baseline mammogram at age thirty-five, to provide a point of comparison for surgeons who may need to operate on the breast later. But few, if any, breast surgeons even glance at the baseline image, because breast tissue changes over the years. For this reason, most health agencies in the United States suggest that a woman's first mammogram occur at age forty. (Most other countries recommend starting later, at age fifty.) It's not that they want to deprive younger women of their God-given right to be radiated! It's just that mammography is not very useful for them. Because the risks from radiation are higher in younger people, repeated early mammography can even be dangerous.

The risk/reward ratio from mammography starts to change somewhere between the ages of forty and fifty, which is when it starts to become more effective—though not as effective as it is in older women. In this age group, mammography cuts the death rate from breast cancer by about 15 percent. That number is significant and important, but it surprises the people who believe that if only more women would get mammograms, breast cancer would be practically wiped out. And false positives in this age bracket are a real problem: If you have a mammogram every year in your forties, there is a 20 to 56 percent chance that you will receive a false positive. For this reason the U.S. Preventive Services Task Force in fall 2009 recommended that most women wait to begin screening mammography until age fifty.

For most women in their forties who do not have a family history of breast cancer, waiting until fifty is fine. If you do have a family history of breast cancer, however, you should consider starting at age forty and having mammograms every year or two thereafter. Family history is usually taken to mean breast cancer in a close relative, but this can be a complicated topic. (If you'd like to learn more about what constitutes a family history of breast cancer and how this is different from the risk of inherited breast cancer, go to www.dslrf.org.)

Recently, digital mammography and MRI have been offered as improvements over conventional mammography, but although they find more "stuff," they don't pass the important test of improving health outcomes. They don't save any more lives, probably because of the biology of breast cancer tumors. Some tumors grow at a moderate rate; these are the cancers for which mammography appears to be most useful, allowing us to catch them before it is too late and treat them successfully. But other tumors are very aggressive and invasive; unfortunately, finding these tumors early has a limited effect on our ability to treat them. Still others grow very slowly and don't always turn into full-blown cancer. A tool that finds more of the fast- or slow-growing cancers may not have a big impact on survival rates, but it will definitely make its owners a lot of money.

Our best hope for beating breast cancer resides not in more imaging but in going beyond it. The story of the cervical cancer vaccine is an inspiration. Here's what Susan has to say:

Thirty years ago, when I was a surgical resident, the Pap smear was established as a screening method for cervical cancer, but the only treatment for an abnormal Pap was a total hysterectomy: tubes, ovaries, uterus—everything. We didn't know what else to do. Most women with abnormal Paps are in their twenties or thirties, so in those days having a hysterectomy often meant losing your chance of having children. A cousin of mine had an abnormal Pap, but she convinced her doctors to watch her closely until after she had a child. Afterward, she had a hysterectomy.

As more research was performed on cervical cancer, we learned that we could respond to the problem locally, with cryosurgery as well as laser and cone biopsies. We also figured out that the first thing to do after an abnormal Pap is to repeat it, because the test can produce false positives. Then it was discovered that cervical cancer was sexually transmitted, and after that we learned it was caused by the human papillomavius (HPV); and now we have a vaccine. Think about the speed of these changes. Thirty years ago, my cousin had a hysterectomy for an abnormal Pap. Ten years ago, my sister had a hysterectomy for HPV. But my college-age daughter has received a vaccine to prevent the disease in the first place!

We made a lot of progress against cervical cancer in just one generation. And we might be able to do the same with breast cancer. Women now get mastectomies for ductal carcinoma in situ (DCIS), which is a condition of the breast that can sometimes lead to cancer. It's like having a hysterectomy for an abnormal Pap. We just don't know what else to do. But we're on the verge of being able to tell which kinds of DCIS lead to cancer and which don't, so we won't have to perform mastectomies on women who don't need them. And then we'll figure out what causes DCIS in the first place. And *then* we'll prevent it. To me, mammography and other forms of imaging are temporary measures that we'll perform until we have something better to offer. The best answer isn't finding breast cancer—or heart disease or osteoporosis or cervical cancer—early on. The best answer is learning how to keep it from happening in the first place.

Where Do You Draw the Line?

A positive development in the world of health screenings is the number of tests that look for risk factors, the signs that tend to appear before a disease develops. In these cases, we really may have the chance to stop a problem before it starts. These risk factor screenings have touched us personally: Susan has high cholesterol and takes medication to keep it under control, and Ali lost weight after discovering that her blood pressure was high.

Keep in mind, however, that risk factor screenings come with a big question: How do we decide that a person's risk is "too high" and therefore in need of treatment? Take blood pressure, for example. Although high blood pressure isn't a disease in itself, we know that people whose blood exerts a lot of force against the vessel walls are more likely to develop coronary artery disease. Blood pressure scores occur on a continuous curve. So do most other risk factors. The higher you sit on the curve, the greater your risk. The position of the cutoff point—the place that divides the people who are at increased risk from the people who are not—is arbitrary. Where the line is drawn depends on the perspective of the person who's holding the pencil. Think of it this way: How do you decide whether you think someone is short or tall? Usually, it depends on your own height. You probably think that anyone who has a few inches on you is tall; anyone who is smaller than you seems short. But a professional basketball player will see things differently.

If you work for a company that manufactures drugs for high blood pressure, your perspective is affected not by your height but by your job. You have an interest in drawing the line as low on the curve as possible, so that more people will feel that they need to buy your product. But if you work for a health insurance company, you might want to set the bar at a higher level, so that fewer people receive coverage for that drug.

Whether to take drugs for blood pressure (or other risk factors) is not a black-and-white matter. The farther down a person is on the risk curve, the less likely she is to receive benefit from any given treatment. The risk of side effects from the drug, however, is the same as for a person who sits at the top of the curve.

What the Health?

Osteopenia (low bone mass) is a new diagnosis that is often called a precursor to osteoporosis (porous bones). But what does osteopenia really mean? The current definition of osteopenia is one standard deviation away from the bone mass of a woman in her twenties. So if you undergo a bone density scan and are given a diagnosis of osteopenia, all it means is that your bones are less dense than a young woman's. No one really knows if this is cause for alarm—no studies have proven that this kind of score is a predictor of fractures—or if it's just a normal part of aging, in the way that it's normal to produce less estrogen or to have gray hair.

When you and your doctor consider whether you should take medication, you have to take into account your family history, the possibility of disease versus the possibility of side effects from treatment, and your own risk tolerance. When you have a risk factor screening, be ready to talk to your doctor about where the treatment line is placed. Be aware that a risk factor is only that: a risk factor. It's not a disease and it's not a life sentence, just as the absence of measurable risk factors is not a guarantee of good health.

How Will the Information Change Your Plan of Action?

If somebody suggests that you have a health screening or any other kind of diagnostic test, ask, "What will you do with the information?" If a test cannot change the plan of action in a useful way, maybe you shouldn't agree to it. If you fall down and injure your rib, you might go to the doctor thinking that an X-ray is in order. In fact, the treatment is the same whether there is a fracture or not—and X-rays are notorious for not revealing rib fractures. In that situation, an X-ray is just extra radiation.

You should also ask yourself whether you're willing to undergo the treatments that could result from the screening process. Because our insurance plans reward doctors for performing more treatments, and because our legal system punishes them severely for missing a problem, it's in physicians' interest to follow up on every oddity that appears in a screening and then to push for medical activity: more screenings, more biopsies, more surgeries, more chemotherapy.

This tendency shows up in a heart-wrenching way in older people who have multiple health problems. An eighty-five-year-old woman in good health, for instance, should continue to get mammograms. But is breast cancer screening wise in a woman of the same age who has many serious conditions and is not expected to live very long? If mammography finds a tumor, does she want to proceed with aggressive and difficult treatment? It's a decision that should by all rights be a personal one, but it can be very difficult to yell "Stop!" at a medical system that defaults to "Go!"

Screening Recommendations

In many cases, the future of health screening is bright, with better and more precise tests in the works, along with procedures that are truly preventive. Until then, we'll have to make the best of what we've got. For the two of us, this means taking a skeptical view of the widely distributed testing schedules we see in magazines and on television shows. Many testing schedules are recommended by groups that have a financial stake in how frequently we are screened. Instead, we like the recommendations made by the U.S. Preventive Services Task Force, an arm of the Agency for Healthcare Research and Quality, which is an independent federal body that bases its suggestions on a rigorous review of published trials. (You can download a free copy of its booklet, the *Guide to Clinical Preventive Services,* at the website www.ahrq.gov/clinic/pocketgd08.) The following are its recommendations for several of the most common screenings. Based on your health history, you and your doctor may reasonably decide to depart from these recommendations:

• **Mammogram:** Women age fifty and older should have yearly mammograms. Women between the ages of forty and forty-nine with a family history of breast cancer should also have mammograms annually. All other women should have mammograms starting at age forty and every couple of years thereafter until they turn age fifty.

• **Breast cancer risk assessment:** Women whose family history suggests an increased risk for breast cancer as a result of mutations in the BRCA1 or BRCA2 genes should see a genetic counselor, who can evaluate them for genetic testing.

• **Pap smear:** Once you have had two or three consecutive annual Paps that are normal, you can wait three years between tests.

• **Skin check:** There is no good data proving that skin checks reduce the risk of death by melanoma, so whether to get an annual full-body skin check is up to you. An alternative possibility is taking advantage of a doctor's visit that occurs for an unrelated reason, and then asking your doctor to be on the lookout for unusual growths.

• **Blood pressure:** Every two or three years, more often if you have high blood pressure.

• **Cholesterol, both LDL and HDL:** Every five years. If you have high cholesterol or other risk factors for heart disease, have it checked more often (exactly how often will vary with the individual). If you do not have risk factors for heart disease and are under the age of forty-five, you can go longer between tests.

• **Colonoscopy:** Every ten years, starting at age fifty. If one of your close family members developed colon cancer before age sixty, or if you have ulcerative colitis, then you may decide to have a colonoscopy before you turn fifty.

• **Bone density scan:** Every ten years, starting at age sixty-five. If you are at a high risk for osteoporosis, you may choose to have a bone scan as early as age fifty.

· **Tests for sexually transmitted diseases:** If you've never been tested for sexually transmitted diseases, or if you have changed partners since your last screening, you should be checked out for chlamydia, HIV, gonorrhea, and syphilis.

From the Trenches...

Recommendations for Pap testing have changed, as we have learned that the HPV virus is the cause of the vast majority of cervical cancer and precancers. As an ob-gyn, I have been less than perfect when it comes to my own gynecologic care. My Pap tests have been done pretty much when I was pregnant or going in for a problem at a gynecologic visit. Luckily, this has averaged out to about every three years. And, wouldn't you know, science has backed up my improvised schedule of Pap testing. This year I went to see my primary care doctor for a preventive maintenance visit, and she suggested I did not need a Pap test since she had done one last year. Hallelujah, said I.

Same thing for breast self-exams. For years I have diligently taught patients the search-and-destroy mission that we know as the breast self-exam. I would do my own breast self-exams when I remembered, from time to time in the shower or when lying in bed at night—certainly not the once a month I was preaching. Then, lo and behold, a study done in China found that breast self-exams are not really doing any good in the early detection of breast cancer and may do some harm in creating more anxiety and extra breast biopsies. Whew. Off the hook again. Now I explain this to patients and tell them to be aware and knowledgeable about their bodies and how they work, and to report anything that seems amiss to their doctor—but no more guilt over irregular breast self-exam schedules.

—*Hope Ricciotti*

Getting Yourself There

You now have a healthy dose of skepticism, loads of questions for your doctor, and an updated, evidence-based set of guidelines on the health screenings most likely to benefit you. But you cannot take advantage of those benefits if you do not show up for the procedures you really need. Doing so can be difficult, especially if you're afraid of what the test will uncover.

One way to face your fear is to say to yourself, "Guess what? If I have a health problem, it's going to be there no matter whether I get this test or not. By getting the test, I'm improving the odds that any problem I have will be caught early on, while it may be relatively easy to treat."

If you fear the discomfort or the ick factor of certain tests, information is also on your side. Ali was the principal investigator of a study that looked at whether relaxation techniques could decrease the pain and anxiety of routine mammograms. She found that the vast majority of women reported mammography caused them little pain or anxiety. Even when some discomfort is unavoidable, it's usually far less painful than having a late stage of the disease you're being screened for. The preparation for a colonoscopy isn't fun—the laxative you have to drink is disgusting, and you have some diarrhea afterward. But it's all over in a day, and compared to having stage-four colon cancer, a colonoscopy is a walk in the park.

When You Get the Call

A few summers ago, Ali went in for a routine mammogram. There were several women ahead of her. The first woman finished up and

Ali could hear the tech call out cheerfully "Bye! Thanks for coming in!" The second woman finished. Again, the tech chirped, "See you next year!" And so on, down the line. Ali had her test and then waited for the tech's happy good-bye. Instead, the tech paused and then said in a sober voice, "Um . . . the radiologist will call you if she sees anything." From that minute, Ali knew she was going to get The Call, the one in which the doctor says, "We may have found something. We need you to come back in."

Most people get a call like this at least once in their lives, and learning how to manage this nail-biting experience is an art. First, you should know that most callbacks do not result in a diagnosis. If you get a callback, go ahead and ask your doctor, "What are the odds this will turn out to be a problem?" It's better to have information than twist in the wind. While you wait to have a second test or to hear your results, know that it's normal to feel jittery. Try to make extra time for relaxation techniques: Write down your fears in a journal; get some exercise; meditate; and challenge any automatic negative thoughts you're having. Don't be bashful about asking for the support you need. In Ali's case, she consoled herself with the statistics about mammogram callbacks, had a couple of anxious nights . . . and then learned that her repeat mammogram was normal.

If you need follow-up appointments and treatments, continue to think about your stress in relation to the resources available to you (see chapter 3). Remember to make a list of things you need and pass it around to the friends and family members who have supported you in the past. They will be glad to help. Wouldn't you be, if your friend were in a similar situation?

And if you are sick and have to deal with the health care system, remember that this is not the time to be a good girl. Susan's cousin once needed to get a test performed urgently, so Susan advised her

From the Trenches . . .

Not too long ago, I went in for a gynecologist's visit and the doctor said she felt a mass on my ovary. So I had an ultrasound, and as the tech was performing it she said, "I don't feel anything; I think you'll be fine." But then my gynecologist kept calling me to talk about the results. I don't know if I was in denial, but I didn't call her back. She tried to reach me several more times.

About two weeks later, I got a certified letter in the mail. It was from my doctor and said, "I've been trying to reach you. I need you to call me right away." And I thought, "Oh, man, I really should have called her and paid attention to this." I called her and, luckily, it turned out to be just a small, benign cyst. That was the first time I ever had to face a diagnostic test. My reaction really surprised me and made me more empathic toward people who avoid hearing what they don't want to know. It made me so sensitive. It's scary.

When you're planning preventive care, you need to know that it might not be enough to go in and get a diagnostic test. When you need to go back, you need to go back. Avoidance and denial aren't therapeutic.

—Janet Taylor

to go to the doctor's office and announce that she would like to have the test performed that day. "I have a book and I have my lunch," her cousin told the receptionist politely, "and I'm prepared to wait all day." The doctor saw her within an hour.

In times of medical crisis, realize that a lot of stress comes from trying to ride a tidal wave of medical information, one that carries you fast. It's difficult to ask clarifying questions and confront the doctor when you're feeling worried or vulnerable. Your partner or mother may feel as nervous as you do, so instead of asking them to accompany you, bring your most obnoxious friend. You know who she is. She will be unafraid to grill the doctor or to ask the same questions over and over again until she understands and can explain things to you later. Just realize that this friend is probably not the same person you'll want to have by your side during a procedure, or have to sit with you while you recover. She'll be too obnoxious!

Chapter Five

It's Not Religion, It's Just Exercise

SUSAN OFTEN JOKES THAT SHE loves to exercise, not because of its health benefits, but because it makes her feel morally superior. Go ahead and laugh (Ali does), but we'll bet you've felt the same way. For many of us, exercise induces the same feelings of righteousness that other people get from going to church—and the sad flip side is that if we don't exercise, we feel morally *inferior*. As two women who have a complicated history with exercise, we'd like to help you separate those feelings of virtue and guilt from physical activity. It's not religion, after all. It's not even a good deed. It's just exercise.

One reason exercise takes on such a moral urgency is that we connect it to another touchy issue: our weight. (In a moment, we'll report some interesting data on the effectiveness of exercise as a tool for weight loss.) Another reason is that exercise is often billed as the ultimate preventive strategy. Work out, goes this line of thinking, and you can avoid nearly every health problem, from heart disease to arthritis. And, in fact, there are hundreds of observational studies showing that people who exercise are healthier in many ways. It's an impressive and exciting collection of data, and one we are sure you've heard over . . . and over . . . and over.

However, we need to interpret these findings with precision, not exaggeration. It's all too easy to jump from "exercise appears to reduce our risk factors for certain diseases" to "exercise has been proven to stop all disease in its tracks" and then on to "if you get sick, it's your own damned fault for not exercising enough." This is where the guilt and pressure come in, and it's why so many women either become obsessed with their exercise regimens or wearily toss up their hands and give up altogether. We believe that by being clear-eyed about exercise—examining its proven benefits, its limits, and where the jury is still out—we can reclaim a happy and healthy middle ground for physical activity.

For starters, exercise is often hailed as a way to dramatically cut your risk of heart disease and certain cancers, including breast and colon cancer. There are several large, well-conducted observational studies demonstrating that people who exercise have lower rates of these diseases. (Remember that observational studies track people's behavior over a period of time, usually through questionnaires, and then try to determine whether people who made one kind of choice are healthier than people who chose differently.) But do these studies prove that exercise is the *cause* of these benefits? Maybe they do, but maybe they don't. People who exercise tend to have other habits that are linked to good health: they eat well, weigh less, and do not smoke. They are more educated and report less stress. The best observational studies try to control for these variables, but it's nearly impossible to completely isolate exercise from the rest of a person's life. So there is still no definitive answer to the question: Does exercise make people healthier—or do healthy people tend to exercise more in the first place?

Without randomized, controlled trials (RCTs) in which one group is assigned to an exercise program and another stays inactive, we won't get the answer. Unfortunately, it's hard to imagine these trials can ever take place, because you'd need the subjects to commit to their program (or to the lack of one) for a very long time to measure the effects on heart disease, cancer, and other problems that tend to surface later in life.

So what's the best way to apply the evidence we *do* have to our daily lives?

This is one of those cases where you have to make a decision based on inadequate evidence. You know how to do this, because, as we've said before, you make these kinds of decisions all the time. When you decide where to live, where to work, and whether to take the freeway or the back roads for your commute, you look at the available evidence, determine its quality, and weigh the risks against the benefits.

When it comes to exercising as a way to prevent heart disease or cancer, what we know is this: There are some good signs that exercise might cut the risk of heart disease or cancer. So the potential benefits of exercise are great. How about the risks? Not bad at all. Exercise has a low side-effect profile—lower than most heart medications—so you're not putting yourself in much danger by working out. (Injuries are real, however. Susan broke her leg while swimming in the rough ocean surf and tore her Achilles tendon while dancing, and you'll read more about Ali's torn rotator cuff soon.) It's this kind of cost-benefit analysis (possible longer life versus risk of injury) that leads the both of us to exercise on a regular basis. But we don't kid ourselves: There are no guarantees.

What about the other supposed benefits of exercise? It's a theory—a promising theory, but not yet a proven fact—that working out could help prevent Alzheimer's disease and other forms of cognitive impairment. Some observational studies have shown that older people who exercise are less likely to get Alzheimer's, but a few other studies contradict this finding. One notable study found that any leisure activity, whether or not it incorporates physical movement, decreases the risk of Alzheimer's. (Interestingly, the only activity that really stood apart from the pack was dancing, whose participants had less cognitive decline than those practicing any other activity. Tango, anyone?) A review of the evidence, published in a 2006 issue of *Neuroscience and Behavioral Reviews,* suggests that exercise may be a potent way to ward off or even treat cognitive impairment—but only in people who do not already have risk factors for cardiovascular disease.

Our verdict? We'll take the educated bet that exercising later in life is good for your brain.

What about weight loss? Doesn't exercise help us take off the pounds? Sadly, most of us do not respond to physical activity by losing a significant amount of weight. An eight-month RCT published in the journal *Archives of Internal Medicine* showed that exercise alone did not lead to weight loss except at fairly high levels of vigorous exercise (jogging twenty miles per week or the equivalent)—and even then, the subjects lost only about 4 percent of their weight. Women especially were unlikely to lose weight on an exercise program that was not combined with diet. This is probably because it's hard to create a large enough energy gap through exercise alone, and also because exercise makes you hungry. While we were working on this book, Susan ran a half marathon with a friend in Florida. She probably burned about thirteen hundred calories. That afternoon, waiting in the airport to fly home, Susan enjoyed a recovery meal of a cheeseburger, fries, and a beer. She deserved every last bite, but she downed more calories in just a few minutes than she burned off during the race.

You can see this as depressing news, or you can try a different perspective. It can be liberating to disconnect exercise from weight loss. This is especially true if you are in the habit of using exercise as a punishment for eating, or as a way to allow yourself to eat "bad" foods. How many times have you heard a woman say something like "I have to run extra miles today because I ate potato chips with lunch"? Now that you know exercise doesn't usually lead to weight loss, you can just relax and enjoy your workouts for other reasons.

These reasons include gaining better mental health and better sleep. So much of the media's attention has been focused on the effects of exercise on cancer or heart disease even though, as we've said, the evidence isn't rock solid. We're less likely to be told about the treasure trove of RCTs that demonstrate the benefits of exercise on mood and sleep. These go far beyond the happy glow that most of us feel after working out. Earlier we described an RCT at Duke University in which exercise was just as effective as medication in reducing depression. This finding is especially compelling because the study focused on moderate to severe depression, and severe depression is often thought to be controllable only with medication.

In a 1998 trial published in the *American Journal of Psychiatry,* panic attack sufferers were randomized into three groups: one took anti-anxiety medication, another group performed cardiovascular exercise, and the third received a placebo. Of all the groups, the exercisers found the most relief from their symptoms. Exercise is also one of the best ways to cope with insomnia. Although no one fully understands the physiology of the sleep-exercise link, several RCTs show that exercise during the day can produce better sleep at night. These results are thrilling to us, because we believe that the goal of engaging in healthy habits is not to live forever. It's to live as long as you can with the best quality of life you can. And here is data showing that exercise can make you happier and help you sleep more peacefully! It's exactly in line with our Pretty Healthy goals.

There is also some excellent evidence that exercise lowers the risk of diabetes. A randomized, controlled study by the Diabetes Program Prevention Group showed that when obese, sedentary people with mildly elevated blood sugar started a walking program, they were much less likely to develop diabetes than people who took blood sugar medications or who did nothing. Controlled, randomized studies have also shown that exercise significantly reduces both pain and disability in people with arthritis in their knees. Yet, oddly, it does not appear to help people with arthritis in their hips, which again makes the point that exercise is not necessarily a cure-all.

In these and many other ways, the evidence for exercise is more of a mixed bag than you may have been led to believe. We let this knowledge relieve our guilty feelings on the days we don't have time to run or cycle. Paradoxically, feeling less guilt about exercise increases our enjoyment of it, leading us to work out more often.

With a more nuanced picture of exercise, you're in a better position to make rational choices about your exercise program. Do you suffer from depression, anxiety, or insomnia? How you treat these matters is a personal decision, but be aware that regular exercise may be able to pull you through a difficult time. Are you obese, with high blood sugar? We hope you'll do something to get moving. (Anything is better than nothing.) Do you have risk factors for heart disease? Even though it remains unclear whether exercise can improve your odds of avoiding cardiovascular problems down the road, it makes sense to try it and know that you're doing your best. (Notice how different this thought is from the frightening and overblown statement "If you don't exercise, you will die of a heart attack.")

Are you relatively young, healthy, physically competent, and very busy? Well . . . for you, it's possible that *not* exercising is a reasonable choice. Susan spent her youth thinking of her body as a carrying case for her brain. She was also busy doing research, working with breast cancer patients, writing books, and raising a family. When she turned age fifty, she realized she was in an age group that put her at greater risk for disease, and she took up running. Now, at age sixty, she runs marathons (albeit slowly—she ran the Boston Marathon and finished a few paces ahead of the guy who juggled four balls the entire way). But does she regret not exercising when she was younger? Not really. She doesn't believe that her current health is negatively affected by the age at which she took up the habit.

A Tale of Two Quizzes

There are not one but two Pretty Healthy quizzes in this chapter: one by Susan and one by Ali. They reflect a fight—er, we mean "energetic debate"—we had over whether it is more important to exercise (to be physically active) or to be fit (to be physically capable, regardless of whether you exercise). It all began when Ali asked Susan to develop a way for readers of this book to quickly assess their fitness level. This is how the conversation went:

SUSAN: Okay. You asked me to come up with a fitness test. I did some research and I've got a good one for us. Here it is: If our readers can walk a mile in twenty minutes, they're pretty fit.

[SILENCE.]

ALI: Um, really? That's all? I know people who could get up off the couch and walk a mile in twenty minutes, but they don't do any exercise at all.

SUSAN: Yeah, but if they can walk the mile in twenty minutes, they're still pretty fit.

ALI: But not pretty healthy.

SUSAN: Why not?

ALI: Because most of the data leans toward the importance of regular exercise.

SUSAN: But the exercise isn't an end in itself. Exercise is recommended because it helps you achieve the *fitness* goal of walking a mile quickly. If you can walk the twenty-minute mile without exercise, that's okay.

ALI: I just can't believe that someone who can walk a mile in twenty minutes is as healthy as someone who can walk a mile in twenty minutes *and* works out several times a week.

SUSAN: Yes, they are! Look at blood pressure, as an example. To be Pretty Healthy, your blood pressure should be 120 over 80. Some people can eat whatever they want and their blood pressure is exactly 120 over 80 . . . and they're Pretty Healthy. Other people make the prescribed changes to their diet, but their blood pressure is still too high. They're not Pretty Healthy. What makes you healthy in terms of blood pressure is not necessarily what kinds of foods you eat, it's having relatively low blood pressure numbers. *The habit is not what makes you healthy.* If you're healthy without following all the health advice, you're still healthy! I think you want health to be more controllable than it is.

ALI: But the papers in the medical journals talk about achieving a certain number of exercise hours, not about achieving a certain level of fitness. Why not?

SUSAN: Inadvertently they *do* talk about fitness. The papers about exercise are telling us what we need to do to be able to walk that mile quickly. And most of the evidence for exercise does not come from randomized, controlled studies. They're observational studies that show us that people who exercise regularly are healthier. But is that because they also go to the doctor more often? Is it because when you're healthy, you tend to exercise more than if you're not?

ALI: But there *are* some randomized, controlled trials that show the benefits of exercise specifically. Look at the depression research, at the Duke University study showing that exercise is more effective against depression than meds. The papers aren't saying that *fitness* is more important than meds.

SUSAN: The research is a moving target, so to speak. The goal is not just to be thin. I think we can say that there isn't a perfect link between exercise and health, but from all appearances exercise is a good idea anyway.

ALI: Let's ask Mim Nelson about this. She's a walking encyclopedia on exercise.

SUSAN: Okay, we'd better ask Mim.

ALI: [Sigh.] I guess you can't get a surgeon and a shrink to agree on everything.

One week later, Ali and Susan talk to Mim Nelson, director of the John Hancock Center for Physical Activity and Nutrition at Tufts University and author of the Strong Women . . . *book series.*

ALI: Here's our question, Mim. To be as healthy as possible, which goal should our readers aim for: to be fit or to have a regular exercise program?

MIM: That's not an easy question to answer. Some of the country's pre-eminent scientists in this field are debating this very question.

ALI: At least we're in good company!

MIM: What I'm going to say is that you're both right. The epidemio-logical studies show that if you are trying to improve your health in terms of risk for cardiovascular disease, diabetes, obesity, all-cause mortality, and, to a degree, bone health, the strongest evidence is that fitness is more important. The evidence is mostly related to aerobic fitness, but some of the findings are skewed because we just don't have enough data on strength training. Nevertheless, the data is really very strong that the risks go down when you are fit, no matter what you weigh or whether you exercise. But the data that looks at the importance of self-reported physical activity is pretty strong, too. It's just not *quite* as strong.

SUSAN: There's a fair amount of overlap in the data, right? It's hard to separate fitness from physical activity in the studies I've seen.

MIM: There *is* a lot of overlap. But when you weigh the evidence, whether fitness or exercise is more important depends on a person's age. Between the ages of twenty and fifty or so, the evidence for fitness is stronger. Yet if people in this age group get enough exercise at a high enough intensity, their cardio fitness is better, their glucose metabolism is better . . . it seems to be a pathway to better health. Now, as soon as you start looking at older adults, fitness may or may not make as big a difference as how much you exercise. That's because other health issues may come into play, things like mental health, depression, sleep, and anxiety. To improve these health problems, just participating in exercise, whether you're fit as a result or not, seems to be helpful. And, in general, there is some evidence that as you go from twenty to thirty to forty to fifty, you have to do more exercise to keep up. You have more to work against as you grow older.

This conversation shows how difficult it is to answer seemingly simple questions about health or to make blanket recommendations for an entire population. Since neither one of us is ready to concede that the other is right, we have each designed our own quiz. The one by Susan is an assessment of your fitness level. The other, by Ali, measures the amount of exercise you get, as well as your attitude toward working out. Put both quizzes together, and do you get the truth about exercise and fitness? Well, maybe. We've given you data and made our arguments. But this is a book about the importance of developing your own conclusions based on the best available evidence . . . so *you* make the final call.

Susan's Quiz: Are You Physically Fit?

I love it when women do triathlons and ride centuries (a century is a hundred-mile bike ride) and perform other hard-core physical activities. But I want to make it clear that the elite level of fitness required for these events is far greater than the amount

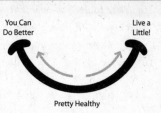

of fitness you need for basic health. It's my bet that you're fitter than you think you are. To prove it, here's a simple assessment. All you'll need are comfortable shoes and a way to time yourself. A wristwatch or cell phone will work just fine.

1. Find a place where you can safely walk for one mile without interruption. A high school track is good, or you can use an Internet mapping tool or your car to measure the roads near your home. When you're ready, walk a mile as fast as you can. Time yourself. Did it take you twenty minutes or less? (If you are unable to walk, you can

(continued)

substitute treading water for twenty minutes or wheeling yourself in a wheelchair for fifteen minutes.)

☐ Yes   ☐ No

2. Now run or jog for a mile. It's okay if you need to jog slowly. Can you do this without stopping? (If the walk in question number one has made you tired, you can skip this question and come back to it another day.)

☐ Yes   ☐ No

3. Stand on one foot. Can you maintain your balance for thirty seconds?

☐ Yes   ☐ No

4. Sit in a chair. Can you stand up without using your arms?

☐ Yes   ☐ No

5. Go to the grocery store and buy what you need for the week. Ask the clerk to put your purchases into paper bags with handles, which hold more stuff than plastic bags. Grab one bag with your left hand and another bag with your right. Can you lift and carry them?

☐ Yes   ☐ No

Scoring

If you answered yes to every question—even if the one-mile run left you gasping—you have demonstrated basic levels of cardiovascular fitness, strength, and balance. You're Pretty Healthy. If you want to get even fitter (and I agree with Mim Nelson—the older you get, the more important this is), the rest of this chapter will show you some easy ways to do it.

If you answered no to any of the questions, read below:

1. The ability to walk a twenty-minute mile is a baseline for physical fitness. Below that line, you're at a much greater risk for disease

(continued)

and disability. If you weren't able to complete a mile in twenty minutes, see your doctor for a checkup to rule out underlying health conditions that may be slowing you down, and get cleared to begin exercising. You can't be Pretty Healthy until you improve your fitness.

2. If you can walk a mile in twenty minutes but can't run a full mile without stopping, you're out of the most dangerous zone, but you could stand some improvement. We'd like every woman to be capable of running a mile, and for plenty of good reasons. You will further reduce your risk of disease—*and* you will be better prepared physically to do things that might save your life, such as run down the steps of a burning building.

3. How do women get bone fractures? By falling down. How do they avoid falling down? By having good balance. If you need some help with balance, you can practice it around the house. Stand on one foot while you hold on to the kitchen counter, or try walking heel-to-toe in a straight line. Or just engage in more physical activity in general, which tends to help you balance for longer periods of time.

4. Getting out of a chair without using your hands is a way to tell whether you have enough leg strength and balance to engage in everyday activities. (You don't want to be the old lady who can't get up and down by herself—you want to be the old lady who can rise up out of her chair and whack an impudent whippersnapper over the head with her cane.) If you answered no to this question, consider a weight-training program. Although weight training is not the only way to get stronger, it has the advantage of allowing you to start with very light weights and work your way up to heavier ones.

5. If you're not strong enough to lift grocery bags, then you're not strong enough, period. A little exercise and/or strength training will increase your muscle power. That way you won't have to depend on the kindness of strangers just to get your groceries into the car.

Ali's Quiz: Are Your Exercise Habits Pretty Healthy?

Read each question and circle the answer that best applies to you. Then tally up your points and read about your score.

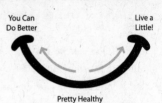

1. How often do you exercise?

0 points. Never.

1 point. On weekends.

2 points. Somewhere between three and six days a week.

3 points. Seven days a week, every week.

2. What do you do if you overeat at lunchtime?

0 points. I skip exercise that day. (Isn't it dangerous to work out on a full stomach?)

1 point. I stick to my normal routine.

2 points. I consider adding an extra day to my workout schedule that week.

3 points. I double my usual routine as punishment for pigging out.

3. When you get sick, what happens to your exercise routine?

0 points. I stop working out completely. If there is anything more disgusting than being sweaty, it's being sweaty *and* snotty.

1 point. I scale back a little, depending on how bad I feel.

(continued)

2 points. If I have a cold, I push through it. With anything worse, I back off and rest.

3 points. You'd have to hospitalize me before I stopped exercising.

4. Which of the following statements characterizes your attitude toward exercise?

0 points. Can we drop the subject? I already know that I'm a bad person for not working out.

1 point. I don't really like exercising, but I do it because I have to.

2 points. Some days I have to force myself to work out, but mostly I enjoy the feeling I get when I exercise.

3 points. It's an addiction. If I miss a workout, I panic.

5. After you exercise, how do you feel?

0 points. Not much different than I did before.

1 point. Like I've earned myself a nice snack.

2 points. I feel good—a little tired but the blood is pumping.

3 points. In serious pain.

6. How would you characterize the intensity of your workouts?

0 points. What workouts?

1 point. Pretty light. I either go for a stroll with friends or I make sure to do things like park my car at the back of the lot and walk from there to my office.

2 points. I usually break a sweat.

3 points. It's not a true workout unless I am groaning in agony.

(continued)

7. Do you warm up, cool down, and stretch as a part of each workout?

0 points. I don't have time for all those things, so I don't exercise at all.

1 point. Nah. I just hit the ground running.

2 points. I try to, although sometimes I cut corners for the sake of time.

3 points. Absolutely! I would never skip it.

8. You're about to work out when a friend calls you and says, "I really need to talk to you right now." How do you respond?

0 points. I don't have the energy for an intense talk. Sorry.

1 point. Sure, let's talk now and I'll work out during whatever time is left.

2 points. Why don't you come with me? We'll walk and talk.

3 points. Maybe later? I have to go running right now.

9. Your partner suggests taking a long hike tomorrow morning. What do you say?

0 points. There's no way I'm getting out of bed early. How about if we grab a pancake breakfast when you get back?

1 point. Okay, but can I join you for just the last half?

2 points. Sure! What a great way to vary my exercise routine!

3 points. Yes, but I'll need to find another time to get in the hour-long run I had scheduled.

Scoring

0–8 points: Depending on your age and risk factors, your low level of physical activity probably puts you outside the PH Zone. If you're in one of those life stages where there is truly no spare time

(continued)

for exercise, don't be too hard on yourself. Just take advantage of exercise opportunities when you can (and see some evidence later in this chapter for the benefits of very short workouts). But if you suffer from chronic exercise avoidance, you have some work to do. See the motivational tips at the end of this chapter. Good luck, and remember every little bit really does count.

9–17 points: You tend to get by with the bare minimum of exercise, but you're still in the PH Zone. Remember that as you get older, exercise becomes more important, so you may need to step up your efforts in the coming years.

18–24 points: You are committed to working out without being a fanatic—which means that you are in the PH Zone!

25–30 points: This score is a cause for concern. When you exercise to the point of serious pain, use exercise as self-punishment, or allow it to become an excuse for ignoring the rest of your life, you are no longer Pretty Healthy. If you can't moderate this out-of-control habit on your own, consider seeking professional help.

Fun with METs

Assuming that you are going to try to exercise regularly, how much is best? The evidence points to a threshold effect, which means that you get the most benefit just by switching from a state of inactivity to a state of moderate activity. If you exercise more than a moderate amount, your benefits continue to increase, but only by a little.

Most experts have settled on a recommendation that is roughly in line with this finding, and they suggest about thirty minutes of moderate exercise on most days a week. Again, the key word here is "moderate." Intense exercise is fine, but it's not necessary. On the other hand, slowly strolling around the block isn't going to cut it, though a slow walk is better than no walk at all. This seems reasonable to us. There's an alternative way of measuring your exercise, however, that we think is more flexible and fun: METs.

A metabolic equivalent (MET) is a nifty way to estimate how much energy you're expending. One MET represents the amount of energy you use just by sitting quietly. Playing the piano uses up approximately 2 METs. Mopping the floor is worth about 3.4 METs, brisk walking expends 5 METs, playing tennis (singles) expends 8 METs, and playing competitive soccer expends 11 METs. The chart on pages 119–125 lists several other activities and their MET equivalents.

The most current evidence on physical activity strongly suggests that expending 20 MET hours per week will provide you the best health benefit. If you walk briskly (at about 4 mph on a flat surface) for an hour you earn about 5 METs. The math is easy:

20 MET hours ÷ 5 METs = 4 hours

That means you'll need to walk briskly for about four hours each week to earn your 20 METs. The fun part is that if you don't want to spend that much time exercising, you can ratchet up the intensity. If you run a twelve-minute mile (stop laughing; that's Susan's pace) you earn 8 METs per hour. Again, let's look at the math:

20 MET hours ÷ 8 METs = 2.5 hours

So you'd need to run for only two and a half hours a week to get the same benefits. Isn't that great? Now you have a real incentive for getting into shape, because if you are able to exercise at a high intensity, you can spend less time working out!

Be careful here, and don't let METs become a source of obsessive thinking. There's no need to time every workout down to the minute and whip out your calculator to be sure you're getting 20 MET

General Physical Activities Defined by Level of Intensity:
The following is in accordance with CDC and ACSM guidelines.

MODERATE ACTIVITY 3.0 TO 6.0 METS (3.5 TO 7 KCAL/MIN)	VIGOROUS ACTIVITY GREATER THAN 6.0 METS (MORE THAN 7 KCAL/MIN)
Walking at a moderate or brisk pace of 3 to 4.5 mph on a level surface inside or outside, such as • Walking to class, work, or the store • Walking for pleasure • Walking the dog • Walking as a break from work Walking downstairs or down a hill Racewalking—less than 5 mph Using crutches Hiking Roller-skating or in-line skating at a leisurely pace	Racewalking and aerobic walking—5 mph or faster Jogging or running Wheeling your wheelchair Walking and climbing briskly up a hill Backpacking Mountain climbing, rock climbing, rapelling
Bicycling 5 to 9 mph, level terrain, or with few hills Stationary bicycling—using moderate effort	Bicycling more than 10 mph or bicycling on steep uphill terrain Stationary bicycling—using vigorous effort
Aerobic dancing—low impact Water aerobics	Aerobic dancing—high impact Step aerobics Water jogging Teaching an aerobic dance class
Calisthenics—light Yoga Gymnastics General home exercises, light or moderate effort, getting up and down from the floor Jumping on a trampoline Using a stair-climber machine at a light-to-moderate pace Using a rowing machine—with moderate effort	Calisthenics—push-ups, pull-ups, vigorous effort Karate, judo, tae kwon do, jujitsu Jumping rope Performing jumping jacks Using a stair climber machine at a fast pace Using a rowing machine—with vigorous effort Using an arm cycling machine—with vigorous effort

(continued)

General Physical Activities Defined by Level of Intensity:
The following is in accordance with CDC and ACSM guidelines. (cont.)

MODERATE ACTIVITY	VIGOROUS ACTIVITY
3.0 TO 6.0 METS	GREATER THAN 6.0 METS
(3.5 TO 7 KCAL/MIN)	(MORE THAN 7 KCAL/MIN)
Weight training and bodybuilding using free weights, Nautilus or Universal-type weights	Circuit weight training
Boxing—punching bag	Boxing—in the ring, sparring
	Wrestling—competitive
Ballroom dancing	Professional ballroom dancing— energetically
Line dancing	
Square dancing	Square dancing—energetically
Folk dancing	Folk dancing—energetically
Modern dancing, disco	Clogging
Ballet	
Table tennis—competitive	Tennis—singles
Tennis—doubles	Wheelchair tennis
Golf, wheeling or carrying clubs	
Softball—fast pitch or slow pitch	Most competitive sports
Basketball—shooting baskets	Football game
Coaching children's or adults' sports	Basketball game
	Wheelchair basketball
	Soccer
	Rugby
	Kickball
	Field or Rollerblade hockey
	Lacrosse
Volleyball—competitive	Beach volleyball—on sand court
Playing Frisbee	Handball—general or team
Juggling	Racquetball
Curling	Squash
Cricket—batting and bowling	
Badminton	
Archery (nonhunting)	
Fencing	

(continued)

MODERATE ACTIVITY
3.0 TO 6.0 METS
(3.5 TO 7 KCAL/MIN)

VIGOROUS ACTIVITY
GREATER THAN 6.0 METS
(MORE THAN 7 KCAL/MIN)

MODERATE ACTIVITY	VIGOROUS ACTIVITY
Downhill skiing—with light effort	Downhill skiing—racing or with vigorous effort
Ice skating at a leisurely pace (9 mph or less)	Ice-skating—fast pace or speed skating
Snowmobiling	Cross-country skiing
Ice sailing	Sledding
	Tobogganing
	Playing ice hockey
Swimming—recreational	Swimming—steady paced laps
Treading water—slowly, moderate effort	Synchronized swimming
Diving—springboard or platform Aquatic aerobics	Treading water—fast, vigorous effort
Waterskiing	Water jogging
Snorkeling	Water polo
Surfing, board or body	Water basketball
	Scuba diving
Canoeing or rowing a boat at less than 4 mph	Canoeing or rowing—4 or more mph
Rafting—whitewater	Kayaking in whitewater rapids
Sailing—recreational or competition	
Paddle boating	
Kayaking—on a lake, calm water	
Washing or waxing a powerboat or the hull of a sailboat	
Fishing while walking along a riverbank or while wading in a stream—wearing waders	
Hunting deer, large or small game	
Pheasant and grouse hunting	
Hunting with a bow and arrow or crossbow—walking	
Horseback riding—general	Horseback riding—trotting, galloping, jumping, or in competition
Saddling or grooming a horse	Playing polo

(continued)

General Physical Activities Defined by Level of Intensity:
The following is in accordance with CDC and ACSM guidelines. (cont.)

MODERATE ACTIVITY	VIGOROUS ACTIVITY
3.0 TO 6.0 METS	GREATER THAN 6.0 METS
(3.5 TO 7 KCAL/MIN)	(MORE THAN 7 KCAL/MIN)

Playing on school playground equipment, moving about, swinging, or climbing	Running
Playing hopscotch, 4-square, dodgeball, T-ball, or tetherball	Skipping
Skateboarding	Jumping rope
Roller-skating or in-line skating—leisurely pace	Performing jumping jacks
	Roller-skating or in-line skating—fast pace
Playing instruments while actively moving; playing in a marching band; playing guitar or drums in a rock band	Playing a heavy musical instrument while actively running in a marching band
Twirling a baton in a marching band	
Singing while actively moving about—as on stage or in church	
Gardening and yard work: raking the lawn, bagging grass or leaves, digging, hoeing, light shoveling (less than 10 lbs per minute), or weeding while standing or bending	Gardening and yard work: heavy or rapid shoveling (more than 10 lbs per minute), digging ditches, or carrying heavy loads
Planting trees, trimming shrubs and trees, hauling branches, stacking wood	Felling trees, carrying large logs, swinging an ax, hand-splitting logs, or climbing and trimming trees
Pushing a power lawn mower or tiller	Pushing a nonmotorized lawn mower
Shoveling light snow	Shoveling heavy snow
Moderate housework: scrubbing the floor or bathtub while on hands and knees, hanging laundry on a clothesline, sweeping an outdoor area, cleaning out the garage, washing windows, moving light furniture, packing or unpacking boxes, walking and putting household items away, carrying out heavy bags of trash or recyclables (e.g., glass, newspapers, and plastics), or carrying water or firewood	Heavy housework: moving or pushing heavy furniture (75 lbs or more), carrying household items weighing 25 lbs or more up a flight of stairs, or shoveling coal into a stove
General household tasks requiring considerable effort	Standing, walking, or walking down a flight of stairs while carrying objects weighing 50 lbs or more

(continued)

MODERATE ACTIVITY	VIGOROUS ACTIVITY
3.0 TO 6.0 METS	GREATER THAN 6.0 METS
(3.5 TO 7 KCAL/MIN)	(MORE THAN 7 KCAL/MIN)

Putting groceries away—walking and carrying especially large or heavy items less than 50 lbs.	Carrying several heavy bags (25 lbs or more) of groceries at one time up a flight of stairs
	Grocery shopping while carrying young children and pushing a full grocery cart, or pushing two full grocery carts at once
Actively playing with children—walking, running, or climbing while playing with children	Vigorously playing with children—running longer distances or playing strenuous games with children
Walking while carrying a child weighing less than 50 lbs	Racewalking or jogging while pushing a stroller designed for sport use
Walking while pushing or pulling a child in a stroller or an adult in a wheelchair	Carrying an adult or a child weighing 25 lbs or more up a flight of stairs
Carrying a child weighing less than 25 lbs up a flight of stairs	Standing or walking while carrying an adult or a child weighing 50 lbs or more
Child care: handling uncooperative young children (e.g., chasing, dressing, lifting into car seat), or handling several young children at one time	
Bathing and dressing an adult	
Animal care: shoveling grain, feeding farm animals, or grooming animals	Animal care: forking bales of hay or straw, cleaning a barn or stables, or carrying animals weighing over 50 lbs
Playing with or training animals	Handling or carrying heavy animal-related equipment or tack
Manually milking cows or hooking cows up to milking machines	
Home repair: cleaning gutters, caulking, refinishing furniture, sanding floors with a power sander, or laying or removing carpet or tiles	Home repair or construction: very hard physical labor, standing or walking while carrying heavy loads of 50 lbs or more, taking loads of 25 lbs or more up a flight of stairs or ladder (e.g., carrying roofing materials onto the roof), or concrete or masonry work
General home construction work: roofing, painting inside or outside of the house, wall papering, scraping, plastering, or remodeling	
Outdoor carpentry, sawing wood with a power saw	Hand-sawing hardwoods

(continued)

General Physical Activities Defined by Level of Intensity:
The following is in accordance with CDC and ACSM guidelines. (cont.)

MODERATE ACTIVITY	VIGOROUS ACTIVITY
3.0 TO 6.0 METS	GREATER THAN 6.0 METS
(3.5 TO 7 KCAL/MIN)	(MORE THAN 7 KCAL/MIN)

Automobile bodywork
Hand washing and waxing a car

Pushing a disabled car

Occupations that require extended periods of walking, pushing or pulling objects weighing less than 75 lbs, standing while lifting objects weighing less than 50 lbs, or carrying objects of less than 25 lbs up a flight of stairs

Tasks frequently requiring moderate effort and considerable use of arms, legs, or occasional total body movements.

For example:

• Briskly walking on a level surface while carrying a suitcase or load weighing up to 50 lbs
• Performing maid service or cleaning services
• Waiting tables or institutional dish-washing
• Driving or maneuvering heavy vehicles (e.g., semi-truck, school bus, tractor, or harvester)—not fully automated and requiring extensive use of arms and legs
• Operating heavy power tools (e.g., drills and jackhammers)
• Many homebuilding tasks (e.g., electri-cal work, plumbing, carpentry, dry wall, and painting)
• Farming—feeding and grooming ani-mals, milking cows, shoveling grain; picking fruit from trees, or picking veg-etables
• Packing boxes for shipping or moving
• Assembly-line work—tasks requiring movement of the entire body, arms or legs with moderate effort

Occupations that require extensive periods of running, rapid movement, pushing or pulling objects weighing 75 lbs or more, standing while lifting heavy objects of 50 lbs or more, walking while carrying heavy objects of 25 lbs or more

Tasks frequently requiring strenuous effort and extensive total body move-ments.

For example:

• Running up a flight of stairs while carrying a suitcase or load weighing 25 lbs or more
• Teaching a class or skill requiring ac-tive and strenuous participation, such as aerobics or physical education
• Firefighting
• Masonry and heavy construction work
• Coal mining
• Manually shoveling or digging ditches
• Using heavy nonpowered tools
• Most forestry work
• Farming—forking straw, baling hay, cleaning barn, or poultry work
• Moving items professionally
• Loading and unloading a truck

(continued)

MODERATE ACTIVITY	VIGOROUS ACTIVITY
3.0 TO 6.0 METS	*GREATER THAN 6.0 METS*
(3.5 TO 7 KCAL/MIN)	*(MORE THAN 7 KCAL/MIN)*
• Mail carriers—walking while carrying a mailbag • Patient care—bathing, dressing, and moving patients or physical therapy	

Source: U.S. Department of Health and Human Services, Public Health Service, Centers for Disease Control and Prevention, National Center for Chronic Disease Prevention and Health Promotion, Division of Nutrition and Physical Activity. *Promoting Physical Activity: A Guide for Community Action.* Champaign, IL: Human Kinetics, 1999. (Table adapted from Ainsworth BE, Haskell WL, Leon AS, et al. Compendium of physical activities: classification of energy costs of human physical activities. *Medicine and Science in Sports and Exercise* 1993;25(1):71–80. Adapted with technical assistance from Dr. Barbara Ainsworth.)

hours per week and not a measly 19.5. If the numbers are making you nutty, think of METs this way: On most days of the week, you should perform either thirty minutes a day of moderate activity—*or* twenty minutes a day of intense activity. Pretty simple. And no matter how you track your exercise, keep in mind that both the thirty-minutes-per-day recommendation and the 20-METs-per-week recommendation are guesstimates, not facts. As with so many other health habits, exercise has a very generous Pretty Healthy Zone.

What's the Least You Need to Do?

This brings us to one of our favorite health themes. Women's lives occur in phases, and some of those phases—especially young motherhood, career building, and caregiving—allow less time for self-maintenance than others. There will be times in your life when twenty to thirty minutes of physical activity is more than you can do in a week, let alone a day. Even our friend Mim Nelson, the exercise physiologist who tried to break our exercise/fitness stalemate earlier in the chapter, admits that she worked out only once or twice a month when her three children were young. "Looking back," she says, "not running for a few years probably saved my joints." Isn't that refreshing? Instead of punishing herself for not exercising much during a busy time of her life, Mim takes a positive view. Now that Mim's children are older, she's back to her regular workouts.

As we see it, the challenge is to enjoy each of life's chapters and to do what we *realistically* can to stay healthy.

You can certainly choose to wait out a difficult time of life, especially if you are young and Pretty Healthy. But don't feel that if you can't get twenty METs per week, your only option is to throw in the towel. Exercise is not an either/or proposition. There are quite a few studies that show a surprising number of benefits to supershort workouts. In one study, sixteen young men, all of whom were moderately active, were randomized into two groups. Over a period of fourteen days, the first group rode a stationary bike for a total of six sessions that lasted between 90 and 120 minutes each. The second group rode the bike at an all-out effort for just thirty seconds at a time, resting or cycling very lightly for four minutes between intervals. They also worked out for a total of six sessions, working their way from four intervals per session to six—meaning that their total workout time came to a grand total of about fifteen minutes over two weeks. Was there a benefit? You bet. Before and after their sprint training period, the study's participants took an exercise endurance test. After sprint training, their endurance doubled, meaning that they were able to exercise at a high intensity for twice as long.

This study is small and looked only at college-aged men, so it's too early to draw definitive conclusions about the benefits of very short but very intense workouts for all of us. But it should give hope to anyone who can't exercise for longer periods of time. We think short-burst exercise is ideal for young mothers, who usually struggle to find more than a few consecutive minutes to themselves, but who could probably sprint across the yard every now and then while playing with their toddlers. Note that we said "sprint," not "lope." The idea is to run as fast and hard as you possibly can. You should be panting afterward.

Other possibilities for short workouts include running up and down the stairs, dashing to the mailbox and back, and doing push-ups while the coffee brews. You'll feel a little batty, but when has that stopped you before? When life allows, you can resume normal workouts.

Reality Check

Do you exercise at a vigorous level for more than forty-five minutes a day, five days per week...no matter what? If so, you are probably enjoying performance benefits from your hard work—but you are not going to see increased health benefits compared with people who exercise less. So if this has been your reasoning, it no longer holds up. Why do you do it then? To become a better athlete? That's great. Because it feels good? We've felt that way, too. Are you trying to punish yourself for eating? Hmmm. That's a problem. Ditto for routinely using exercise as a way to escape your obligations at home or work.

Fussy Fitness Rules

One of the fitness culture's most tenacious myths is that if you're not adhering to a series of strict rules about how to exercise, you might as well not exercise at all. You've heard these rules, or variations on them, a million times. We're all supposed to warm up for five to ten minutes, hit a specific heart rate and maintain it for at least thirty minutes, cool down for five to ten minutes, do balance work, *and* stretch for five minutes—otherwise, we've blown it.

Fortunately, our bodies aren't really this finicky about how we treat them. They are capable of getting fitter under many circumstances, not just a few narrowly prescribed ones. Can you imagine if the cavemen knew about these fitness "rules"? There they'd be, running after a woolly mammoth, when one caveman would stop and say, "I've got to slow down! If we run any faster my heart rate is going to exceed the fat-burning zone." And another would say, "Time out! I'm about to go anaerobic!" Humanity would never have evolved past *Homo habilis,* because we'd have been too busy monitoring our heart rates to chase down dinner. Eventually we would have grown so weak and slow that the woolly mammoth would have eaten *us.*

A better guide to rely on when you're working out is your own common sense. Take the target-heart-rate zone. According to the charts you see in gyms across the country, there is an ideal range for your heart rate while you're exercising, calculated according to your age. Go below that range, and you won't get health benefits. Go above that range, and you're courting danger. Trying to stay in this zone can drive you bonkers, because those charts don't take into account the wide variability of heart rates from one person to another.

You don't need those charts, as you have more experience with your body than any chart ever could. *You* know when you're working hard, when you're pushing yourself to your very limit, and when you're coasting. And as for the fat-burning zone, the math doesn't work. Yes, you burn the highest percentage of calories from fat when you keep your heart rate between 60 and 65 percent of your maximum ability—but if you work at a higher intensity, you burn a higher number of calories total. So liberate yourself from heart-rate charts and silly exercise rules, sisters, and make your own decisions about the intensity of your workouts.

As for the importance of warm-up and cool-down sessions: Warming up is good because it appears to reduce the risk of injury, and cooling down helps because it allows a gradual return to normal blood flow and heart rate, but, honestly . . . if you're a basically healthy person there's no need to be a fanatic about it. When you're engaging in a vigorous activity or one that has you making sudden or unusual movements, a warm-up and cool-down make good sense. But when you step outside for a brisk walk during your half-hour lunch break, you don't need to devote ten or fifteen of those precious minutes to warming up and cooling down. Both of us tend to jump right into our exercise routines, though Ali prefers to cool down toward the end, to avoid that unpleasant hot-and-sweaty-while-showering feeling.

Let your body tell you how gradually to ease into and out of whatever exercise you're doing. One caveat: If you have heart disease or other serious health problems, or if you are elderly, then you really are at a greater risk of injury or circulation problems, so you should definitely follow the warm-up and cool-down advice.

Balance work isn't necessary unless you actually have trouble balancing or are frail and more likely to injure yourself if you fall. If you need to improve your balance, there are several ways to go about it. Exercise of all kinds tends to increase balance, so if you are inactive, get moving in whatever way you enjoy. If you are age sixty-five or older, you may benefit from exercise that is directly intended to

---

Uh . . . *Duh!*

A study has proven what every woman has known since the dawn of Jazzercise: Music improves your workout. In a study at Hampden-Sydney College in Virginia, volunteers who rode exercise bikes while listening to music pedaled faster than those who rode in silence. So next time you exercise, don't be shy about breaking out your favorite tunes (and if you wear headphones, no one needs to know you're partial to "Sweatin' to the Oldies").

---

increase balance. Yoga, tai chi, ballet classes or videos, or just practicing your balance at home are all good choices.

Finally, there's stretching. Stretching doesn't have a lot of evidence in its favor, but a little flexibility tends to make you feel more comfortable. Certainly, being *in*flexible can hamper your mobility and even be painful. It seems smart to stretch at the end of your workout, while your muscles are warm, but there are some people who feel that they are less prone to injury during exercise if they stretch gently beforehand. Your call.

What About Strength Training?

ALI: I have a disaster story about strength training, in which just about everything went wrong.

I work full-time, I have two young children, and I'm working on my sixth book. I don't have a lot of time. I walk—fast—several days a week, but I've always felt that I should also lift weights. So I asked around about a strength-training website to help me perform the exercises correctly. I got the name of one, settled in one evening to exercise, and then the website crashed. I figured out how to download an instructional video from the Web, but it didn't work. Mim Nelson actually called the company for me and they mailed the video to my house. The video arrived in January . . . and it stayed in the carton for the rest of the year. Literally. That New Year's Eve, I resolved (again) to start weight training. I chose Tuesdays and Thursdays as my weekly training times.

The first Tuesday of the new year, I actually opened the carton. I got out my husband's hand weights. I started watching the video and discovered that I was supposed to have a towel, a chair, and some ankle weights. I found a towel and a chair, but I didn't have ankle weights. So I fast-forwarded through the ankle weight exercises and started at the free-weight section. Unfortunately, I tore my rotator cuff a few years ago and it turned out that Dave's weights were too heavy for me. I did the exercises, but then I couldn't move my shoulder for the next six days.

Eventually, my shoulder felt better, so I went to the store and bought a box of ankle weights. And the box is still sitting next to my bed, very close to where the video carton had sat unopened.

I'm so frustrated. I'm worried that I've been a bad role model for my daughters, because I haven't done what I said I would do. Any ideas?

SUSAN: You have a seven-year-old, right? And I know you—you carry her around a lot, don't you? There's your weight training, right there.

ALI: You're right! Katie's my Velcro kid, always attached to me; I carry her around all the time. I feel *so* much better now.

We do tend to get hung up on the details, don't we? Ali spends most of her working life helping other people solve their problems, yet here she couldn't see the forest through the trees. It's another case of being a little bit brainwashed by the fussy fitness rules—in this case, the one that says the only way to get strong is to lift hand weights. But of course there are many ways to increase your strength; it's just that formal weight training is the easiest strength exercise to measure in controlled studies, and so formal weight training is what makes the headlines.

Also, it's easy to get confused about the purpose of being strong. First and foremost, we want you to be able to carry your groceries, shovel snow, and raise your garage door by hand when the remote breaks. When you can't do those things, you lose some of your independence. Obviously, this tends to be more of an issue as you get older. When you're younger, you may naturally have enough strength to meet life's challenges—unless you are seriously sedentary or overly thin, in which case it's possible to be twenty-five and still be as weak as an old lady. In these situations, some kind of strength training can help.

Another reason women are told to lift weights is that studies have shown weight training increases bone-mineral density. This is true, but it's not the whole picture. The idea behind this advice is that by increasing bone density, we can avoid osteoporosis and disabling fractures—yet there is more to osteoporosis than bone density. We don't yet understand all the factors that contribute to osteoporosis, but it's clear that the quality of the bone is also important, as are the bone's micro-architecture, your overall weight (being thin is the number one predictor of osteoporosis), and genetic factors. You don't want to go into menopause with weak bones if you can help it, but you also can't store up extra bone density when you're young and then "spend" it when you're older. Furthermore, fractures in old age aren't usually caused by osteoporosis itself. Poor balance, weak eyesight, and medications that make you dizzy are the leading causes of falls.

So if you are weak, there are plenty of good reasons to get strong. And if you enjoy weight training, go for it. But if you engage in real-life weight training (children, garage doors, sacks of mulch), you're Pretty Healthy just as you are.

Getting Past Good Intentions

The two of us hate gyms. We don't like being told how to work out and we feel stupid in the workout clothes we feel pressured to wear. (No matter what the catalogs say, stretchy yoga pants are *not* flattering to all body types.) The point is not that gyms are bad; we know plenty of women who enjoy them and who get great workouts there. The point is that we've all got our hang-ups when it comes to exercise, and if you are trying to start or improve an exercise routine, acknowledging those hang-ups is important. The psychological literature tells us that when it comes to making a change, willpower alone isn't enough. You also have to anticipate obstacles and find a realistic way to integrate the new behavior into your existing routine.

With that in mind, here are ten of our hard-won tips:

· **Exercise is like flossing your teeth—if you do it at the same time on the same days each week, it will become a habit.** This is why every morning at 7:15, after her older daughter has left for the bus stop, Ali hops on her recumbent exercise bike and rides until 7:45, when she has to get ready to take her younger daughter to school. If you don't have a regular schedule, do what Susan does and spend a few minutes each Sunday previewing the week ahead and figuring out how to fit in exercise. Then write it into your calendar.

· **If your life is unpredictable, you need exercise that's portable.** Walking and running are great for travelers because all you need to pack are clothes and a pair of running shoes. Ask the concierge or anyone at the front desk for a good, safe route to take. Many hotels keep trail maps on hand.

• **Exercise with a friend.** You are more likely to get out of bed and work out when you know your friend is waiting for you at the bottom of your driveway. Ali much prefers walking with a friend than walking alone, because if she's busy chatting she doesn't notice that she's walking up a murderously steep hill. Although Susan is a dedicated lonesome runner, she does like being part of a group that meets before and after a run.

• **Anticipate sabotage.** It sounds cynical, but other people can get so uncomfortable when you make a change that they will try to stop you. Ali recently mentioned to a friend how proud she was of being able to cycle ten miles in thirty minutes on her stationary bike—and the friend said, "Oh? But have you lost any weight yet?" It's the kind of comment that can deflate you in an instant. So be prepared for sneak attacks as well as "supportive" sabotage, such as "Honey, you don't need to work out. You look great already!"

• **Hitch yourself to a star.** You remember star charts . . . you know, where a kid gets a star sticker for each time she cleans her room or gets dressed by herself? They're a powerful tool for shaping behavior. Grab on to some of that for yourself by keeping track of your exercise achievements. Make your own or use one of the widely available online tools, such as www.onlinefitnesslog.com. Susan, a gearhead, has a watch that tells her the pace and elevation and everything else about her run. When she gets home she can upload the data to her computer and compare one run with another, which helps her stay motivated.

• **Have a goal.** Become determined to run a 5K or a half marathon, or to ride your bike up the hill without stopping. Tell *everyone* about your goal and when you're going to achieve it. Your pride won't let you back down. Plus, you'll get to hear people tell you, "Wow! You did a great job!"—a phrase you may not hear often enough now that you're a grown-up.

• **Embrace disco.** It's more fun to exercise when music is playing. There are websites, including www.podrunner.com, where you can choose the exact intensity of your workout (135 heartbeats per minute, 160 bpm, and so on) and then download music that matches it. The selections lean toward techno music and electronica, though, so if that's not to your taste you can always download recordings from an online music store and create your own workout mix.

• **Keep things lively with sprint training.** When Ali read the journal articles touting the benefits of short duration / high intensity exercise, she wondered if her own workout might benefit from sprints. Now she spends twenty seconds out of each minute on her stationary bike pedaling as fast as she can. She's noticed an increase in her stamina as well as a side benefit: The varied pace makes her workouts fly by.

• **Mix it up.** Remember how we said in the stress chapter that variability in your heart rate is good for you? We believe that's true for your entire body—and your mind as well. So if you started a walking plan six months ago because you couldn't dream of getting your reluctant body to run . . . well, maybe now you're fit enough to try a walk-run mix. Or you can go hiking. Or swimming. Change thwarts boredom, which is the great enemy of good habits.

• **We've noticed that a lot of you forget to** *choose an activity you enjoy.* Give yourself the time to try out a few things and discover what's truly fun. Start with the activities you liked when you were younger. Ali knows a woman who hated to exercise until she remembered that she loved to roller-skate when she was little. Now she goes in-line skating at the park on her lunch break. But don't be afraid to

Why Do You Work Out?

Susan works out because when she has grandchildren, she wants to be able to lift them into the air and take them down the playground slides on her lap. Ali works out for the mood lift: No matter how bad she feels when she starts, she feels better when she's done. We asked some of the other BeWell Experts about their motivation to exercise:

To feel better about my aging body. I get energized and mentally clearer after I sweat. Also, I now realize that not having physical exercise is not an option for me.   —Janet Taylor

I want to live longer and healthier. I may not be able to be thin, but I am able to be strong. I don't want my muscles to atrophy and discover that lifting suitcases has become a thing of the past! I always feel better afterward, too. Even if the trainer has reduced me to a bowl of jelly, I am a happy bowl of jelly.   —Pepper Schwartz

I work out because I want to be able to keep walking and feel good. I had forgotten what feeling good felt like.   —Byllye Avery

To have fun. As we get older we start perceiving movement as a "stress rehearsal" rather than a joyful experience. No child acts as if going out to play is a punishment. Maybe we should hire children to be our personal trainers!   —Loretta LaRoche

To feel strong and energized, and in touch with myself.
                                                   —Chris Economos

Because it improves my quality of life. I'm happier when I'm active, I sleep better, I can eat more good food, I'm less stressed, and I feel that I am doing something good for myself. And I work out because I want to live for a long time and enjoy life to its fullest. Sounds corny, but it's all genuine!
                                                     —Mim Nelson

try something completely new. Maybe you felt slow and pokey when you ran laps in gym class . . . and maybe now you are still slow and pokey but very, very persistent, which makes you a perfect candidate for a marathon. There are plenty of team sports for adults, including softball, volleyball, and even dodgeball. If you enjoy competition, there are masters clubs for people over thirty-five who want to swim, row, do track and field, and many other activities. And the great news is that the competition starts getting scarcer in middle age, so you have a better chance of winning!

Chapter Six

Eating Well: Beyond Blueberries

I N H E R B O O K *The Blessing of a Skinned Knee,* psychologist Wendy Mogel describes the ancient Jewish belief that God will hold us accountable at the end of our lives for all the good foods we were offered but chose not to taste. Times have changed, food is much more abundant than it used to be, and if we adhered to this philosophy literally we'd all be as big as Hummers. We love this principle, though, because it reminds us that life should be pleasurable, and that delicious foods—including crisp french fries and hot fudge sundaes—are gifts we should savor.

We need this reminder because it's hard to enjoy food if you believe it is either medicine or potential poison. Yet isn't that what most of us do? We've been taught that by eating precisely one cup of blueberries per day, we can dose ourselves with enough anti-oxidants to ward off Alzheimer's. That one glass of red wine will roar through our poor clogged arteries like liquid Drano. Or that a croissant can stop our hearts as instantly as if we were electrocuted. So instead of saying, "What's cooking? Smells great!" we poke at our skinless chicken breasts like forensic detectives, asking, "How much fat is in this?" Or we pop baby carrots joylessly, as if they were pills.

We want you to have fun with your food again. Take blueberries, for instance, which used to be a summer treat best enjoyed in luscious pies or cobblers. More recently blueberries have received attention for their supposed ability to prevent heart disease, so now this seasonal delight has become a chore. If you attend a Manhattan power breakfast at any time of year, you'll see tables full of slender executives dutifully eating their bowls of raw berries, which look sadly naked without their cloak of buttery cobbler topping. You have to wonder what these diners are thinking. Maybe, *Gee, these little guys taste much better—not so rubbery—when they're in season and have a little sugar sprinkled on top . . . but at least now I'll live forever.*

There is, in fact, some evidence that blueberries can lower cholesterol, as reported in the article "Effect of Blueberry Feeding on the Plasma Lipid Levels of Pigs" in the *British Journal of Nutrition,* but that evidence is slim. The article details a study in which a group of pigs was fed a diet that included pulverized dried blueberries. A second group received an identical diet, minus the berries. When the pigs were given blood tests, it was revealed that the blueberry group had lower cholesterol levels.

This finding is interesting, but . . . hello? *Pigs?* Producing an effect in an animal or in a petri dish is much, much different—and often much easier—than producing one in actual live people. And, oh yes, the study was funded by a not-so-surprising source: the blueberry industry.

The next time you hear a claim about the power of a food to heal you, prevent disease, or give you instant cardiac failure, take one of those deep, cleansing breaths you learned in yoga class. Ask yourself: Do I know the details of the study? Was it conducted on humans? Who paid for it?

We've noticed that "superfood" studies tend to align themselves according to predictable patterns. We just described one of the patterns, which is to show an effect in an animal or in the laboratory, but not in people. Another strategy is to demonstrate that the food in question contains a substance that has already been associated with health benefits. There is already plenty of good evidence that anti-oxidants are good for you, so all that the blueberry industry has to do is demonstrate that blueberries contain antioxidants and, *whoosh!*, we are flooded with a tidal wave of news about the cancer-fighting, artery-clearing, mind-blowing powers of blueberries. Never mind that you can also find antioxidants in each of these foods:

Blackberries	Spinach
Carrots	Strawberries
Kale	Sweet potatoes
Mangos	Tomatoes
Purple grapes	Watermelon

And nearly every other fruit and vegetable.

With all the competition in the antioxidant department, it's no wonder that blueberry growers would want to fund a study of their crop, which is fairly expensive and might not seem all that appealing next to more moderately priced fruits and vegetables.

Another pattern of "superfood" evidence occurs when research-ers take a longitudinal study, one that has gathered lots of information about many people's health habits, and retrospectively mine that data for evidence that healthy people ate more of a certain food. If the two of us wanted to prove that banana-nut pancakes were health foods, we might look at data collected by the Nurses' Health Study. This study's original mission, which was to study the long-

---

From the Trenches . . .

I like to push myself at work. When I have a big project to do, like writing a grant proposal or submitting a paper for publication, I can multitask and stay focused and handle an incredible amount of stress without using brownies or ice cream to console myself. But there's a price to pay afterward.

After you send in a grant application, there's no immediate feedback. You wait for months to hear whether you've received the grant. Or after you submit a paper for publication, you wait for months to find out whether the paper's been accepted. And so I don't experience a celebration when my work is done, because I don't know whether the work has been successful. It's more of a letdown. That's when I get into a funk, and I tend to eat too much ice cream or way too many chips with guacamole.

During these letdown periods, I try to ride things through and put my less-than-perfect nutrition in perspective. I understand that it's all right to indulge in some treats or get a massage or have something done for myself. It brings me back into balance.

If you can keep your head on straight during these nutritional ups and downs, you can stay healthy. But if you get panicked and worried when your routine is thrown off, it can be really dangerous, because you feel like you're on a roller coaster all the time.

—*Chris Economos*

term consequences of oral contraceptive use, has expanded to include the role of nutrition in chronic diseases. Every four years, about one hundred thousand women in the study fill out a food frequency questionnaire. The two of us could comb through these questionnaires, looking for women who had eaten banana-nut pancakes, and try to determine whether they had fewer heart attacks or cancers than women who did not. Like the other two methods, this approach is not illegitimate, but it's not conclusive, either, because the study wasn't designed to test this particular question and doesn't provide a good means of control.

So if you like blueberries, that's fine with us. They're not medicine, but like other fruits, they are good for you. The only time we've ever seen blueberries cause negative side effects is when Violet Beauregarde, of *Willy Wonka and the Chocolate Factory,* chewed on blueberry-flavored gum and swelled into a blueberry balloon. As scientists, we can firmly say that there are decent odds that this will not happen to you. But if you'd rather eat fresh tomatoes or strawberries, don't feel guilty about *not* eating blueberries.

The Big Picture

If you can't rely on media reports about foods that are good for you (or bad for you), how do you know what to eat? This may sound like a rhetorical question. Don't we all know what's good for us? As the two of us began thinking about this chapter, we thought this was so. We said to each other: *Good nutrition is just common sense . . . lots of fruits and vegetables, whole grains, lean protein, and low-fat dairy.* It's so clear. So easy.

And then we turned to the research, confident that our biggest problem would be managing the teetering stacks of papers that proved our assumptions. We were sure we'd be drowning in a sea of high-quality data, of large-scale studies that randomly assigned people to different kinds of diets, controlled for variables, and proved clearly that our "commonsense" diet resulted in vastly improved health outcomes.

Soon, it became clear that we would have to begin a new diet, one whose featured entrée is a heaping helping of crow. We were correct about the stacks of papers, because there really are tens of thousands of studies out there about almost every conceivable aspect of nutrition. Often these studies represent meticulous work by excellent scientists, and they make useful contributions to our body of knowledge. But as far as we can tell, only *one* diet has been studied for its health effects on a large, basically healthy population, using control groups and randomly assigning people to either one kind of diet or another. This is the DASH diet ("DASH" stands for "Dietary Approaches to Stop Hypertension"), and we'll come back to it very soon. First, though, let's talk about why there is so much less gold standard evidence than we expected, and how to make decisions based on the evidence that *is* available.

Why isn't there more proof for our "commonsense" diet? You can guess the first answer: money. It's wildly expensive to recruit hundreds of people to take part in a long-term study; randomly assign them to one of two or three diets; take their health measures before, during, and after the study; and hire staff to oversee the entire operation. Even if this kind of study were within the financial reach of more scientific institutions, analysis of the data poses even bigger challenges. For example, how could the study's investigators be sure that the subjects actually complied with their diets? Most studies rely on questionnaires to measure food intake, a method that is notoriously unreliable. (Can you imagine being asked to recall how many servings of nuts you ate over the past six months? And if you were asked, "How many servings of sweets do you consume in an average week?" could you imagine telling the truth?) And because everyone has to eat, it's very hard to understand exactly what effects you are measuring when you change someone's diet. If a person is healthier when she eats more fish and whole grains, is this because of the fish? The whole grains? Or because she gave up fast food to eat the fish and whole grains? Nutrition is a puzzle with thousands of moving pieces.

And yet, despite our surprise and disappointment at the lack of gold standard evidence for nutrition, neither of us felt comfortable saying, "Okay, eat whatever you want. It doesn't matter." Because what you eat *does* matter. People with risk factors for type 2 diabetes are much less likely to develop the disease if they reduce their intake of fat and calories and increase their intake of fiber. Eating more fruits and vegetables and fewer foods that are high in fat is a known way to reduce high blood pressure. Eating too much of anything can lead to obesity, especially for people who are vulnerable to weight gain, and obesity is linked to a myriad of health problems.

This is the state of nutritional affairs: We know that food affects health, but we do not yet know exactly which diet or diets is best for us. This leaves you (and the two of us) in a situation that by now should be familiar: You'll have to make your decisions based on incomplete information. Although there is less evidence that you or we might want for one specific diet—*much* less evidence that you might suspect for low-fat diets or low-carb or low-salt or high-protein diets—there are many studies, both large and small, that point toward a very broad pattern of eating that is associated with better health.

This means that you don't have to worry so much about whether you should be eating Tibetan yak's milk cheese (for its omega-3s) or if it's better to spend your calories on orange juice supplemented with calcium. Nor will you have to focus your energy on exorcising a single nutritional demon. (Sugar? Saturated fat? Trans fat?) Instead, you can focus on nutrition's big picture, which consists of wholesome, fresh, real foods. This happens to describe—oh, hallelujah!— the foods we identified earlier: lots of fruits and vegetables, fish, nuts, legumes, whole grains, lean protein, and low-fat dairy.

What is so reassuring about this big picture is that it is not a faddish new thing. It's been around for decades (in the world of nutrition science, the equivalent of millennia) and is summarized in two slightly different eating plans: the DASH diet and the Mediterranean diet.

The history of the Mediterranean diet is worth tracking, and not just because it suggests a healthful way of eating. Thanks to an overly simplistic interpretation of the diet by the people who set nutrition policy, the disastrous low-fat food craze was born. Since we would like to avoid eating repulsive products like low-fat sour cream and low-fat mayonnaise ever, *ever* again, let's spend a few minutes understanding how anyone came to believe that such things could be good for us.

The Mediterranean diet came out of Ancel Keys's famous Seven Countries study, which was performed in the 1960s and aimed to understand why the incidence of coronary heart disease was so much lower in southern Europe than in northern Europe. Keys analyzed the dietary patterns of different population groups and discovered something you and I know very well: People everywhere like to eat fat. (Uh . . . *duh!*) He also made a more surprising discovery. The people in the north, where heart disease was prevalent, got their fat from dairy and lard. People in the south, where heart disease rates were much lower, ate olive oil, nuts, and fish.

This might have seemed like a mere coincidence except that Keys also performed controlled-feeding studies, in which subjects ate only those meals that had been specially prepared for them, and showed that people who ate more saturated fat had much higher levels of cholesterol than people who ate more polyunsaturated and monounsaturated fat. As a result, there was a big push in the 1960s and 1970s to change the types of fat eaten in countries such as the United States and Great Britain—and heart disease rates were cut in half. Most likely there were additional factors at work as well, but switching good fats for bad fats was clearly a significant aspect of the improvement.

In the 1980s, however, something changed. The public health message emphasized getting rid of all fat, not just saturated fat. Walter Willett, chair of Harvard's nutrition department, says in an article in *Public Health Nutrition,* "The origin of this policy is somewhat hard to determine, but many nutritionists apparently believed that individuals would find it too difficult to understand the different types of fat and that it was easier just to tell them to reduce all fat, even though the goal was to reduce saturated fat. This policy appears to have had no empirical basis, as it could well be easier to substitute one type of fat for another than to reduce fat in the diet." Gee, you think? Anyone who has ever tried a radically low-fat diet knows how unsatisfied and hungry it makes you feel.

The result, as Willett describes, was the energetic marketing of unappealing nonfat products, repeated advice to satiate your appetite with loads of pasta and bread . . . and the beginnings of an obesity epidemic. At about the same time, the nationwide decline in heart disease began to slow.

Since then, the facts about fat have reemerged, but a lot of damage has been done. You probably know someone who lives in fear of the fat in olive oil, salmon, or nuts, even though research has shown that these fats can increase HDL, which is the good kind of cholesterol that protects your heart, as well as lowers triglycerides. We've also learned that trans fats are especially bad, because they can raise LDL, the "lousy" cholesterol, while lowering HDL. You can go a long way toward improving your diet just by replacing processed foods, which tend to be high in trans fats, with nuts and heart-healthy oils.

The Mediterranean diet encourages people to make this kind of change, along with following the other patterns in traditional Mediterranean cuisine: fruits and vegetables, grains, fish, and moderate amounts of wine. Although each of these foods is known to have benefits, the good health enjoyed by the people who follow a Mediterranean diet probably has more to do with how the different elements of the cuisine come together, and almost certainly with the fact that the diet avoids highly processed foods. (And you absolutely can't rule out nonnutritional factors such as genetics and stress levels in the Mediterranean region.) All in all, it's a very pleasant way to eat, and maybe this contentment helps account for the healthy hearts of the Mediterranean people.

The Mediterranean diet has a lot in common with the DASH diet. The DASH eating pattern may feel a little more familiar to Americans: fruits, vegetables, grains (mostly whole grains), lean poultry, meat, and dairy. A rigorous controlled-eating trial showed DASH to be effective at reducing blood pressure, especially when sodium intake was limited, and a prospective study of thirteen thousand graduates of the University of Navarra in Spain concluded that people who followed the DASH diet had a much lower incidence of type 2 diabetes than people who followed the typical American diet.

There are some differences between the DASH and Mediterranean plans, though. DASH encourages low-fat dairy and more meat, while the Mediterranean diet puts more emphasis on nuts, olive oil, fish, and wine. Both eating plans have good evidence behind them, and individual elements of the plans (such as eating plenty of vegetables) are backed up by some of those other smaller or less well-designed trials that may not mean a lot on their own but that, cumulatively, add up to a convincing pattern. Chances are that if you put the Mediterranean diet and the DASH diet together in a way that fits your needs and suits your palate, you'll end up with a Pretty Healthy way of eating.

There are many places where you can read about the details of each plan, including exactly how many servings to eat of each food group, but we'll spare you the pain. Those details are there for the researchers who need to be explicit about their findings and for people who need to sell diet books. You have no need for them—because, really, it's all about a general attitude toward food.

The Mediterranean diet, for example, is based on observations of the way people eat over time, not what they consume every single day. Although most versions of the Mediterranean diet suggest eating one to two servings of fish each week, don't panic if there is a month when you don't eat fish at all. It's not as if anyone has proof that a moderate deviation from the diet will cause harm. And yes, the official DASH diet recommends four to five servings of vegetables per day, but as far as we know no one has run a study showing that people who eat a measly three servings per day are less healthy.

We'd rather look for more opportunities to enjoy good meals than spend precious brain cells keeping a tally of how many portions of fish and vegetables we've eaten each day or week. There are diet gurus who love to tussle over how many eggs to eat per week (Two!

None! One hundred!) or whether it's better to drink milk or take cal-cium pills . . . and while these matters are legitimate areas of research, we've seen too many women become so distracted by the hubbub around one single food, or the debate over a particular number of servings, that they lose sight of the big picture. Let's say it again: fruits and vegetables, whole grains, lean meats, beans, fish, nuts, low-fat dairy, and moderate amounts of wine.

Oh, brother, you're thinking, *I knew this already!* That's our point. You have probably been on this earth for somewhere between twenty and ninety years, and you have this nutrition stuff down cold. You know about fruits and vegetables and low-fat or skim milk and whole grains and quality meats in reasonable portions. You know that you should put a variety of colors on your plate (the yellow pep-pers and the green broccoli and the brown rice and the bright red tomato sauce) and that you should shop around the edges of the gro-cery store, where the freshest food is stored. You know that crunchy is good (fiber!) but foods advertised as "crispy" are probably deep-fried. You know that on some days you will eat too much junk food out of stress or fatigue or sheer love of raspberry-flavored Fig New-tons. You even know that there will be *whole weeks* out of your life when the going is really, truly rough—whether you are preoccupied with final exams or a pipe bursts in your kitchen just as your children come down with the flu—where you will survive solely on pizzas washed down with premium ice cream. And that is okay. You will weather these storms and you will go back to your routine of eating wholesome foods in moderation.

What you really need to do now is turn down that jabbering in-ternal voice, the one that distracts you from what you know, deep down, about eating. This is the voice that tries to get you to believe that a healthy diet involves magic tricks, as in: *Well, there was this ex-*

Uh . . . Duh!

In June 2000, the journal *Neurology* published an article demonstrating that doing cocaine while drinking a lot has even more negative effects on cognition than doing either one separately. This study may be useful for the doctors who study addictions, but did the rest of us really need science to explain that cocaine and alcohol—whether together or apart—aren't brain foods?

---

pert on television who said that cabbage is the key to weight loss or *If I eat twenty-five grams of fiber daily, I won't get colon cancer and then I can skip my colonoscopy* or *I can eat Crisco by the spoonful as long as I don't have any carbs.* When this kind of chatter starts up, it's time to channel a person in your life who is calm, kind, and reasonable. Your mother? (Stop laughing.) Your sister-in-law? (Seriously! Stop laughing!) Your fourth-grade teacher? Whoever it is, stop, take a deep breath, and imagine this person saying—in a loving but amused voice—"Oh, you know better than that!" And you do.

What About Weight?

Imagine that when you're born you're given a car, the one car you will have for the rest of your life. You have no say over what make or model you get. You might end up with a Mercedes convertible, a MINI Cooper, or a VW bus. You'll drive your car to high school and to your first job. If you have a baby of your own, you'll bring him or her home from the hospital in the car's backseat. Later in life, someone may use the car to drive *you* to your retirement home.

And if by chance your car is in an accident or if the bumper falls off . . . then, oh well. You'll have to reattach the bumper, live with the dings, and do whatever else it takes to keep your car going, because you'll never get another one.

Do you sense a metaphor coming? Your body is like that car. No matter what the magazines and diet books say, you can't trade in your dependable station wagon for a sleek Jaguar. Or your sweet little MINI Cooper for a muscular sport-utility vehicle. Although you may take some hits along the way, you were born with a basic shape. It was part of the deal when you arrived on this planet, no do-overs allowed.

You were also born with a genetically programmed weight range. Some nifty research has demonstrated this fact for us. In her book *Rethinking Thin,* the *New York Times* science writer Gina Kolata describes two studies performed by Ethan Sims, a scientist at the University of Vermont, in the 1970s. Sims recruited prisoners to voluntarily become fat by eating as much as they wanted. Monitoring the men as they stuffed themselves with up to ten thousand calories per day, Sims expected them to gain weight rapidly—but he was stunned when it took them somewhere between four and six months to become obese. This was much longer than anyone had expected. Sims then found a reason for the men's relative difficulty gaining weight: When the men increased their caloric intake, their metabolisms accelerated by up to 50 percent. Then Sims found a group of extremely obese men and had them diet until they reached the same weight as the now-heavy prisoners. This second group needed half the number of calories to maintain their weight as the first group did—which, you will surely agree, is completely unfair. *Half* the number of calories for the exact same weight! At the end of the study, the newly obese prisoners went back to their normal eating patterns and easily returned to their previous weights.

"Calories in, calories out," chant the diet books, implying that all people burn calories at the same rate. According to this theory, big people are big simply because they eat so very much more than their slender counterparts—and weight gain is inversely proportional to the amount of a person's self-control. But Sims's studies, and others like it, suggest this is not necessarily the case. It's far more likely that each of us has a genetically programmed weight range of about ten to twenty pounds. One person's natural range might be from 160 to 180 pounds, while another's might be from 115 to 130. Yet both people may eat the same number of calories and perform roughly the same amount of exercise.

Where we are within our range depends on our habits, and this is where those lifestyle choices really do have an effect. When we eat less and are more active, we're closer to the bottom of our personal range. When we eat more and are less active, we're at the top. Because we live in a world of abundant, cheap food, many of us are on the heavier end of our range. Our genes make it challenging for us to get much bigger or much smaller. That's why it was so much work for Sims's prisoners to become obese. (But if we eat way too much for way too long, even those of us who are naturally slender can blow the ceiling off our weight range and become obese. This happens when we, like Sims's prisoners, stop listening to whether our bodies are actually in need of sustenance and start cramming in calories like crazy.)

Your goal is not to compare yourself to another person's body shape but to determine your own Pretty Healthy Zone for nutrition and weight. No matter whether you are naturally slender or naturally robust, you want to avoid the extremes of your weight range and find that happy middle ground. You get there by eating good food in reasonable portions. No overly restrictive diets and no gluttony. (Do we really need to tell you that obesity is associated with profoundly

What the Health?

It's a truism that eating a variety of foods is good for you, but you'll get a good laugh out of what most people's dietary variety scores actually measure. "Many people have high scores on dietary variety questionnaires," says Mim Nelson, "but only because they're eating a variety of junk foods. They're eating Snickers *and* Twinkies *and* Doritos." So don't assume that a diverse diet automatically equals a healthy one.

higher levels of mortality from a variety of scary health problems, including diabetes, heart disease, and cancer? Or that starving yourself isn't such a great idea either?)

Caution: Your personal Pretty Healthy Zone for weight—the middle of your range—may put your body mass index (BMI) into the overweight category. There is a brilliant solution to this problem: Ignore it. A study by the Centers for Disease Control found that overweight people tend to live longer than those in the obese or normal categories, which makes us wonder: If most of the population is in the overweight class for BMI, and if being overweight can lead to a longer life, isn't it time to find a less pejorative name for this category? How about "average" . . . or "Pretty Healthy"?

Moderation: It's the New Extreme

Often in this book, we have the pleasure of making the point that the healthiest choices are the easiest to make, because they're nestled comfortably between two extremes. It's really not hard to locate the middle road that leads to Pretty Healthy sleep, Pretty Healthy stress levels, Pretty Healthy exercise, and Pretty Healthy relationships.

But food . . . ah, well, we won't lie to you. Pretty Healthy nutrition is all about delicious, wholesome foods in moderation, but in our food culture, moderation is hard. And eating mostly wholesome foods can be *really* hard. Try counting the number of times in just one day that someone offers you a processed, highly sugared treat, whether it's at the drive-through ("Would you like a chocolate chip muffin with your coffee?"), at the school drop-off ("Please welcome our new school nurse with doughnuts in the gym!"), at work ("It's Karla's birthday; be there for cake and ice cream at three o'clock!"), and at home ("Honey, my client brought us this huge box of chocolates and no one at the office wants them . . . do you?"). It is excruciatingly unjust. Even if we ignore half the consumption messages that bombard us daily, we'll still be eating way too much junk food.

That is why gimmick diets are so alluring. Diets that tell you exactly what to eat or that place entire categories of foods off-limits take personal choice out of the equation. Instead of having to weigh the individual merits of each food offering, you can turn off your brain and say, "No, sorry, can't have that muffin. . . . I'm on that new diet, the one where you stimulate your metabolism by eating nothing but Fritos." If you're going to be Pretty Healthy, you have to find a way to stand confidently in front of our culture's massive smorgasbord and select foods that will truly nourish you.

We're not telling you this to deflate your spirits. We just want you to understand what you're up against. If you want to follow a moderate, reasonable, enjoyable eating plan, you will need the strength to resist temptation—and you will also need to know when to give in to it. This may mean that you'll have to reject the chocolate chip muffin, the school doughnuts, and the office birthday cake, but maybe enjoy a few pieces of chocolate before sending the rest of them to the garbage heap.

With practice, moderation becomes easier. (Susan maintains that moderation comes with age; she swears that in her fifties she lost her taste for sweets. Ali is still waiting for this miraculous development.) You may have already discovered this for yourself; we certainly hope that many of you no longer see yourselves as "problem eaters" but as women of healthy weight who eat the right things most of the time. But it's possible that even with our forgiving definition of Pretty Healthy nutrition, you may stand outside of the PH Zone—maybe because you are obese or because even with a reasonable weight you eat far too much junk food. Or perhaps you have become hypervigilant about proper nutrition and can no longer enjoy your food. No matter what the circumstances, we'd like to help pull you back into the PH Zone. You can start with behavioral changes that will make it harder for you to mindlessly overindulge and easier for you to slow down and really enjoy your food. Many of the following ideas originate from the work of Brian Wansink, a Cornell psychologist whose book *Mindless Eating* describes his findings about the triggers that lead to overeating:

Sit down at a table to eat. Snack food manufacturers spend millions of dollars trying to get us to eat on the couch or in the car, because they know that in these environments we will eat more food of lower quality.

Eat with other people. Sharing meals with friends and family increases your enjoyment—and the shame factor prevents you from going back for thirds.

Seek out smaller plates and silverware. Most plates and utensils made in the last decades are freakishly oversized, tricking us into eating larger servings than we'd normally consume. Wansink's studies have found that even nutritionists will unwittingly help themselves to larger portions when they use big plates and utensils. If you can't find attractive dinnerware of normal size at the store, try going to estate sales or garage sales for vintage pieces.

Don't get cozy with the serving bowl. People eat 30 percent more food when a serving bowl is on the table. Try leaving the bowl on the countertop or by the stove. Similarly, there ought to be a warning label on chips and cookies: Do not eat directly from bag!

Don't eat anything that is labeled "low fat." This is the Snack-Wells Effect. Not only are low-fat versions of normal foods less tasty, Wansink's studies show that people routinely—and unconsciously—eat much more of a product when the "low fat" label is affixed to it. Instead, eat normal food in normal portions.

From the Trenches . . .

When you're a surgical resident, you run all day long. You eat at weird hours, and you catch meals when you can. You learn to live on peanut butter and crackers, because that's what's around. Yet you live through it.

Now that phase of my life is over and my diet is much better . . . but I am addicted to gummi bears. I'm talking about the good ones, Haribos. I eat so many of them that the other day I had to have a come-to-Jesus session and finally forced myself to look at the package label. I realized that I've been eating nine hundred calories a day of nothing but cellulose and sugar! When I go through the day eating a few gummi bears here and there, I find that by bedtime I've eaten a whole bag. So I will have to change the habit. [*Long sigh.*]

—*Nancy Snyderman*

Quiz: Are Your Eating Habits Pretty Healthy?

When it comes to food, we can all be a little wacky at times. That's fine, as long as you avoid the extremes of seeing food as either a devil or substitute for love. To find out if your food attitude is Pretty Healthy, circle the statement that most closely describes

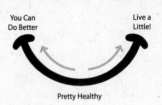

how you feel. Then tally up your numbers and read about your score.

1. How often do you weigh yourself?

0 points. Never. I won't even go for a checkup because I don't want to step on that scale.

1 point. I weigh myself only when my clothes start getting tight.

2 points. Once or twice a week.

3 points. Every single day.

2. How closely do you follow a healthy eating plan (fruits and vegetables, whole grains, lean protein, good fats)?

0 points. I don't even try. My diet consists of crispy things that come in brightly colored packages.

1 point. When life goes according to plan, I eat pretty well, but if my kids get sick or I have a tight deadline, healthy eating goes out the window.

2 points. Most of what I eat is healthy, but if a brownie crosses my path I'll eat it without guilt.

3 points. I do not waver from my healthy eating plan. To be sure I'm on track, I measure every single gram of food that goes into my mouth.

(continued)

3. How often do you diet to lose weight?

0 points. What did you say? I couldn't hear you because these potato chips are really crunchy.

1 point. I usually cut back on my portion sizes after the holidays.

2 points. When my clothes start getting tight, I'm more careful until I get back to my baseline.

3 points. I've never *not* been on a diet.

4. When you decide it's time to change your eating habits, how do you prepare yourself?

0 points. I'm so far gone I've stopped trying to change.

1 point. I think about it for a day or two. Sometimes I make changes as a result, and sometimes I don't.

2 points. I ask myself whether now is really a good time to change and then figure out what I can realistically do to alter my eating habits.

3 points. I implement severe dietary restrictions immediately; no preparation necessary.

5. When you go to a fast-food restaurant, what do you order?

0 points. Whatever is cheesy, meaty, and fried.

1 point. Fast food is a treat for me, so when I go, I make a point of enjoying the house specialty, whether it's a Big Mac or a Burrito Supreme.

2 points. I try not to each much fast food, but I do like a good burger now and then. I try to order apple slices instead of fries, though.

3 points. If I am forced to enter a fast-food restaurant, I whip out my emergency ration of arugula salad and Luna bars.

(continued)

6. When you go to a nicer sit-down restaurant, what do you order?

0 points. What *don't* I order?

1 point. I have either an appetizer or dessert, but not both.

2 points. Something that looks fresh and in season; something I find appealing and enjoyable.

3 points. No bread, no salt, hold the sauce. Then I eat half the food and pour black pepper over the rest.

7. If you have a craving for a treat, how do you respond?

0 points. By pulling one of the candy bars out of my purse.

1 point. I wait to see if the craving passes. If it doesn't, I indulge it.

2 points. I eat a small portion of something really good, like dark chocolate or salted nuts.

3 points. I stand in front of a full-length mirror, grab my thighs, and shriek, "Fat, fat, fat!" until the craving subsides.

8. Where do you eat your meals?

0 points. I plop down on the couch, park a bag of food on my belly, and flick on the tube.

1 point. I eat breakfast and dinner at a proper table, but lunch is usually at my desk.

2 points. At the kitchen table, mostly.

3 points. Wherever I can be alone. I don't like other people watching me while I'm eating.

9. You've overindulged at lunch. What do you do?

0 points. Squelch the guilt by eating even more at dinner.

1 point. Try to accept that when I'm stressed out, food is my tranquilizer of choice.

2 points. Eat a light dinner and forget about it.

3 points. Exercise for as long as it takes to burn off the extra calories.

(continued)

10. Every Hershey's Chocolate Kiss comes wrapped in foil, with a thin sheet of white paper protruding from the top. What are the words on the paper?

0 points. "Stop Reading and Eat the Damned Chocolate"

1 point. "Kisses, Kisses, Kisses"

2 points. "Chocolate Contains Beneficial Antioxidants"

3 points. "The Number One Cause of Death in the United States Is Heart Disease"

Scoring

0–9 points: Well, we have to give you credit, because your answers are obviously honest! But you are not in the PH Zone for nutrition. For whatever reason, whether it's stress, lack of time, lack of attention, or something else entirely, you are eating without thinking. You need to achieve more balance in terms of what you put on your plate and into your mouth. More fruit, fewer chips. More nuts, less peanut brittle. More seltzer, less soda. However, don't feel too glum, because many of us have been there before. The rest of this chapter is full of ideas for making realistic, steady changes to your eating habits.

9–14 points: Despite the craziness of our food-and-diet-obsessed world, you've managed to hold on to a Pretty Healthy enjoyment of food. Although you may wander away from good nutrition when you are under stress, you usually return to your healthy eating habits when life returns to normal. You're in the PH Zone, and that's something to celebrate! But if you ever find yourself in a long-term crisis, you may need to find alternate ways of managing your stress load.

15–21 points: Congratulations on having a remarkably sane food attitude that lands you in the PH Zone. You love to eat, but you also know when to say when. After dinner tonight, toast yourself with

(continued)

a glass of bubbly. Chase it with a Hershey's Kiss, whose wrapper says—as you probably know—"Kisses, Kisses, Kisses." Pure poetry.

22–30 points: Two words: Lighten up!—and we're talking about your attitude, not the number of calories on your plate or the numbers on your scale. Your extreme attitude prevents you from taking joy in your food, and it probably leads to quite a bit of unhealthy stress. Until you stop seeing food as something that can hurt you and start thinking of it as a source of pleasure, you won't be in the PH Zone.

Let only the good stuff into your home. This tip comes from Chris Economos, who notes that it's hard to eat well when we're out in the world: "That's why it's so important to make the home a healthy environment. You won't have to feel so bad about eating what you're served at a meeting if you know that you have control over what you eat at home." (On the other hand, Ali likes setting an example of moderation for her kids by keeping junk food in her home—but eating it at a reasonable pace.)

When Even Small Changes Are Too Big

Food is such a touchy issue, so charged with emotional energy, that for some people even small changes, such as changing where you eat, can be overwhelming. If this describes you, don't give up just yet. Take heart from the work of James Prochaska, the director of the Cancer Prevention Research Center at the University of Rhode Island. He has devoted his career to investigating how people successfully implement new health habits. He's discovered that change is not a single, sudden event. It occurs over time, sometimes lots of time—and it involves a lot of what Prochaska identifies as the "contemplation" stage. From the outside, the contemplation stage looks like a whole lot of nothing, but it may actually be the most vital part of the change process. During contemplation, a person undertakes a realistic appraisal of the pros and cons of change, along with an assessment of the obstacles ahead. At this point, she may decide on a plan for overcoming those obstacles—or she may legitimately choose to postpone change until another, more appropriate time.

If you're considering some changes to your eating habits, you may feel the urge to start right away, but maybe it's wise to mull things over first. Is this a good time to rock the boat? Do you have a new baby, a sick parent, a work crisis, or financial troubles? If you do, maybe it's better to wait awhile. Otherwise, you may be setting yourself up for failure, which can discourage you from trying again later.

When you decide that the time is right to develop a plan—even a plan that consists of small, easy steps—consider it from every angle. The less chaos in your life, the better your chances are of making a realistic and effective change. But there are exceptions. Sometimes one kind of change can lead to another. If you are about to start a new job in a new city, kick things off at the new office by packing a healthful lunch or resisting the urge to set out your usual bowl of mini candy bars for passersby.

Ask yourself: Who can I count on as an ally? How can I handle any sabotage that might come my way? A partner or a close friend who feels threatened by your new habits is going to make things more difficult for you. On the other hand, if you have a weight-loss buddy or an exercise partner, you'll increase the odds of sticking to a new plan.

If you have made other successful changes in the past, what has

The Crap Factor

I wish nutrition labels could be revised so that they offer information that is really useful. For example, they could tell us how many real fruits and vegetables are in the product. And there should be a Crap Factor. You could look at it and it would tell you much crap—how much processed junk—is in the food. That would make food choices a lot simpler.

—*Mim Nelson*

worked for you? What have you learned from previous attempts that were unsuccessful? A few months ago, Ali read a great book called *Secrets of a Former Fat Girl*. The author, Lisa Delaney, lost seventy pounds and kept it off for twenty years by taking very small steps toward improving her habits. At one point, Delaney came up with a mantra called "It's Not an Option," or "INO" for short. Every time she saw a rich food, Delaney would say to herself, "INO," and walk past it.

Ali wanted to drop a few pounds herself, so she decided to give the INO approach a try. Her first opportunity came when she saw a bowl of potato chips sitting on the counter.

"INO," Ali said to the potato chips. "You are not an option."

She turned her back and began to walk away when she heard the potato chips sing out, "Oh, yes we are!"

And so Ali learned from experience that INO was INO for her own weight-loss plan. Instead, she thought things over and tried again. Now she has found that keeping healthful snacks, such as pre-washed carrots and grape tomatoes, in the fridge has helped her make better choices.

Maintenance: The Final Frontier

Prochaska's work on change also has an interesting take on the final phase in the change process: maintenance. It's widely believed that the vast majority of dieters do not maintain their weight loss. Recent research shows that the compliments dieters receive when losing weight are highly motivating, but when those compliments start to fade after the goal weight is reached, dieters start to put the pounds back on. If you want to maintain your positive changes—whether you are trying to lose weight or simply eat more healthfully—you will need to find some ways to continue the positive reinforcement long after people stop saying, "Hey! You look great!" You'll have to find a way to applaud yourself for performing a really hard job well. Think of ways to reward yourself on a long-term, continual basis, maybe with inexpensive but attractive clothes, or with extra time for yourself at the end of the day. Or perhaps you have a goal that really sets you on fire. The two of us have become highly motivated to eat well because we are older mothers and want to live long enough to meet our grandchildren and watch them grow up. Other women have enjoyed being nutritional role models for their families.

Whatever you do, don't let your goal of better nutrition turn into a war with your body. Yes, you want to be healthy, and *we* want you to be healthy. But as the two of us grow older, physical changes are taking place that remind us to love what we've got. Susan doesn't like noisy restaurants anymore because it's too hard to hear what her dinner companions are saying; Ali finally acknowledged on her fiftieth birthday that she needed reading glasses (after her niece observed that Ali's arms were "not long enough to read the menus"). You'd think we'd be sad about these signs, but actually we've noticed that our bodies have started to feel like a favorite pair of old jeans; even if we aren't tall and blond, we can relax into ourselves like never before. We keep trying to eat well, and we exercise, but somehow we're less obsessed with the idea of perfection. And maybe that's the definition of Pretty Healthy moderation.

Fat versus Sugar

We asked the BeWell Experts the eternal question: Which is worse—fat or sugar?

SUSAN: Sugar has gotten a bad name. Everything is blamed on sugar, but it's not an evil in and of itself.

MIM NELSON: Well, sugar is more problematic than fat, but only because it's in *everything* these days.

SUSAN: That's true. I stood in the grocery store the other day and couldn't find a single box of cereal that didn't have added sugar, except Uncle Sam.

CHRIS ECONOMOS: Both sugar and fat are bad in excess.

ALI: But there are healthy fats . . .

MIM NELSON: And there aren't healthy sugars or sweeteners.

NANCY SNYDERMAN: But, really, is there such a thing as bad food? Eating *anything* occasionally isn't going to harm you.

CHRIS ECONOMOS: Deprivation is the root of overeating. We don't want people to totally deprive themselves and boomerang into overindulgence.

MIM NELSON: You know what? This is a dumb question. Everyone knows that the answer is irrelevant. Both are bad if you eat too much, and both are fine in moderation. Next!

Chapter Seven

You, Me, Us: Healthy Relationships

SOCIAL SUPPORT IS ONE OF the key indicators—and possibly a key driver—of health. Yet a poll by the National Sleep Foundation shows that 40 percent of women respond to overwork and stress by cutting back on the time they spend with friends and family.

Right here, right now, let's debunk the idea that friendship is a luxury. Over and over, studies have shown a strong relationship between social support and longer life. One study in Sweden followed seventeen thousand men and women and found that having strong social ties was associated with fewer deaths during the study's six-year period. The study factored in the subjects' initial health status as well as age, gender, education, employment status, and smoking, drinking, and exercise habits. In a Japanese study of six hundred people, also controlled for demographic variables, people who lived alone were more likely to be in poor health compared with people living in extended families.

The studies we've just described are observational studies, the kind that analyze long-term patterns of behavior and their effects on health. Usually we try to bring you the kind of randomized, controlled trials (RCTs) that set the gold standard for scientific inquiry, but there aren't that many RCTs when it comes to relationships and health. It's impossible (or certainly unethical!) to randomly assign one group of people to have a lot of good friends and another group to submit themselves to long periods of social isolation. So we have to rely mostly on observational studies, and it's important to acknowledge that these show only an association between having a supportive social network and being healthier or living longer. They don't show cause and effect. Perhaps the people in these studies who appear to benefit from having close relationships also practice other health habits that may reduce their risk of disease and increase their chances of living longer. Or maybe the road runs in the other direction. Maybe it's good health that allows people to socialize and make friends.

Social scientists have found a few clever ways to run some controlled trials in this field, however, and the results back up what the observational studies have found: There are health benefits to friendship. In two studies published in the *British Journal of Psychology,* a group of chronically depressed women were randomly assigned to receive a voluntary "befriender" or were placed on a waiting list for one. The befrienders were instructed to become confidantes of the depressed women and meet with them regularly for coffee or go on outings together. Seventy-two percent of the befriended women experienced a remission in their depression, compared with only 45 percent of the women in the control group. In another clinical trial at the University of Pittsburgh School of Medicine, 166 people were recruited either alone or with three friends or family members to receive treatment for weight problems. The participants were assigned to either a standard program of diet, exercise, and behavioral modification along with social support, or to behavioral treatment alone. At the end of the four-month study and at a ten-month follow-up, people who signed up for the study along with their friends and family had lost more weight than people who came to the study alone. The social support component of the treatment also had a positive impact, especially when combined with having friends and family aboard during the study. Those who were recruited with friends and given both behavioral treatment and social support were much more likely to stay in treatment and maintain their weight loss.

So it appears that having close friends and family helps us lose weight, fight depression, and live longer. The most widely accepted reason is that social support buffers the negative impact of stress. Caring friends and family members may also encourage us to practice good health habits, such as complying with medical regimens or exercising. But beyond the data, we want friends and family in our lives not just to make us healthier but to improve our human experience. Friends bring us laughter, connection, and, if we're lucky, homemade chocolate chip cookies. When we return these favors, friendships allow us to cultivate our own capacity for generosity.

That said, some relationships can be bad for both your health and your soul. Relationships that include physical abuse or mental cruelty are bad news, obviously, but social damage has more subtle forms as well. In a 2007 study at the University of Missouri at Columbia, young women who talked excessively with peers about their problems—revisiting their troubles every day, even when nothing new had happened—experienced a rise in cortisol, a stress hormone. In other words, hanging out with people who encourage you to dwell on your problems could actually make those problems worse.

You also have to beware of "catching" your friends' bad habits, such as smoking or drinking too much. One Harvard study, using an analysis of thirty-two years of data from the famous Framingham Heart Study (again, this is an observational study, but it's the best we've got), concluded that people with obese friends are more likely to become obese themselves. And friends who dole out unwanted advice and admonish you to get over your legitimate problems may contribute to your stress, not alleviate it. The effects of harmful friendships are made worse if these relationships are so consuming that you miss out on chances to develop more positive friendships.

Of course, no woman in her right mind would read these study results and immediately drop a good friend who happens to be obese or talks too much about her problems. Studies can't tell us everything we need to know about friendships. We'd prefer that you gauge the health of your social support system by looking at the full range of your relationships. And, most important, look at the level of giving and taking that's going on between you and your friends. The best sign of a positive, healthy social network is a basic level of reciprocity. Are you getting what you need socially? And are you giving back in return? It might be that your friends offer you support on a day-to-day basis, but in times of crisis you come sailing through for them. Or maybe you do most of the physical help, like having a friend's kids over to play or hosting her family for dinner, but she might offer support that's more emotional (she's a good listener) or even material (she lets you use her summer house for vacations).

Remember the premise of this book: For every aspect of your life, there is a large Pretty Healthy Zone. In your relationships, there should be some giving and some taking, but don't get stressed about finding a balance that is absolutely perfect. Some women are naturally inclined toward giving. They love to throw parties and listen to people's problems and help those in need. They may give more than they receive, but if they derive pleasure from their activities, they can definitely be Pretty Healthy. In fact, if you're one of these natural givers, it may not be realistic or healthy to expect everyone else in your life to give back to you as much as you choose to give out. Ali, for example, bakes about twenty birthday cakes a year for her friends. She loves baking and she loves making her friends feel special. But does she expect everyone to reciprocate? No. She would be setting herself up for disappointment. (She'd also have a *lot* of cake to eat every May.) As long as your needs are being met, it's fine to have more weight on the giving end of the scale. You may even find that you seek out people who need you, because together you make a good match.

But if you take a good, hard look at your social circle and realize that you are continually being sucked dry by the people around you, it's time for something to change. (At the end of this chapter, the two of us develop an action plan for this circumstance.) And if you suspect that you take more from a friendship or romantic partnership than you give, don't abuse the other person's good nature. Find an equilibrium that works for both of you, or you risk losing that person altogether.

What's the First Thing to Go?

We asked the BeWell Experts: When you are overworked, what's the first thing you cut from your schedule?

CHRIS ECONOMOS: Sleep.

NANCY SNYDERMAN: Sleep and exercise, which is so stupid because exercise is the one thing that can bring me back to normal.

HOPE RICCIOTTI: I don't give up anything. I eat *more!*

MIM NELSON: Exercise. When I'm busy, the time crunch is not just a perceived problem. It's real. But then I come out of it and have time to exercise again.

SUSAN: I don't stop running because I sign up for road races ahead of time—and then I have to do them because everyone's expecting me to be there. But I do give up playing the piano, which I really love.

ELIZABETH BROWNING: I tend to keep exercising because I make appointments with my trainer. But I give up doing things with my friends.

ALI: Time for myself. I love reading the newspaper every night, but that's one of the first things to go when I have too much to do.

Relationship Challenge: The Caretaker Needs Taking Care Of

It's one thing to say that friendships, romantic partnerships, and other relationships ought to be healthy. It's another to know what to do when a relationship hits a bumpy spot. The two of us brainstormed how to handle four of the most frequent relationship challenges for women. You can read the results throughout this chapter; below, we toss around the problem faced by women who are used to assisting their friends and family but are now in the position of needing help.

ALI: A lot of women give and give. And when a crisis happens, they're *still* giving to other people, until they are bled dry. I have patients who are going through demanding infertility treatments and who are also trying to care for their parents and take care of their friends' problems. For many of them, it's the first time in their lives that they need to focus entirely on themselves—but everyone in their world still expects them to give all their energy and time. Susan, you have probably seen women with breast cancer who have this problem.

SUSAN: Well, even though theoretically you're supposed to stop and take care of yourself during a major crisis and allow other people to take care of you, for some women maybe it's better to keep up the role of giver. When things go wrong it can be too much to change who you are. I'll tell you something similar that happened to me: When I was a resident, my sister died. It was totally out of the blue—she fell out of a tenth-story window. It was a shock.

ALI: Oh, my God.

SUSAN: When I got the phone call at work, another resident noticed that something was really wrong and asked if I wanted a hug. I said no . . . and I finished my rounds. Even though working at a time like that probably seemed inappropriate, I needed to do what I knew how to do, which was work. I knew that later I could go and deal with my feelings. In the same way, the person who takes care of everybody will still take care of everybody through her own crisis, because that's just the way she does things.

ALI: But I have a story that counters your point. A few years ago, I had a patient who had just finished treatment for breast cancer: chemotherapy, radiation . . . her ordeal was finally over. And I asked her, "Why are you starting psychotherapy now, after you've been through it all?" She said, "During chemo and radiation, I was so amazing—I went to work every day, I cooked every meal, I helped my family and friends. But now I've hit a wall. It took an enormous toll on me to maintain my normal life through treatment, and I can't keep it up anymore."

SUSAN: See? Psychologically, she needed to keep going during treatment. When it was over, *then* she could collapse.

ALI: But the price she paid for keeping it all together was too high! She came to me because she needed someone else's permission to turn her attention inward. She told me she wished that she had come to see me months ago, because she needed support in learning to meet her own needs and to say no to others without guilt. I use her story as an example when I talk to cancer patients about stress management, because if this woman could do it all over, she would take more time for herself during her months of crisis and not push herself over the edge.

SUSAN: I still think it can be comforting, at least initially, to say, "Even if my body is turning against me, damn it, I can still do my thing."

ALI: I agree that you should keep doing the things that make you feel better. But drop the things that don't!

SUSAN: Yes. Some women have to keep going to work because it's part of their identity, but they don't need to take the dog for a walk or do the school carpool. They can get other people to do those things.

ALI: If you are the rock for everyone and now you are in a crisis, there are a lot of people who owe you. It's time to cash in your IOUs. And if you ask somebody to help you and she says no, but doesn't give a really good explanation or offer to help in some other way, it means two things: One, you move on to the next person on your list, and two, you aren't going to offer your help to that person again. I worry about relationships in which one person is always giving and the other is always taking.

SUSAN: Especially if you are feeling bad about it. Sometimes you know you're being used, and it's okay anyway.

ALI: There's a difference between helping and being used. Helping is good, but being used is *never* okay.

SUSAN: What's the difference?

ALI: Helping is when you willingly do something to improve the quality of someone else's life. When people make it appear that they need more assistance than they really do, you're being used. Women who get used a lot are probably women who are also good at being helpful. Maybe it was their role as a child. Older daughters especially tend to be mommy's helper.

SUSAN: That's me! Especially when you're the oldest child in a big family, as I was, it becomes your job to take care of everyone else.

ALI: I'm used to helping, too. A friend of mine lost his father last week, and even though I had just returned from a business trip and was about to leave on a book tour, I spent Sunday night baking banana bread for him. It made me feel good to give my friend something of my own making. There was a lot of love baked into that batter! People say to me, "How do you keep on giving? How do you keep your own cup full?" But giving in that way fills my cup. It makes me feel really good.

SUSAN: That's what I was trying to say earlier. If being a giver is part of your self-image and one of your roles in life, giving that up can make you feel worse. When you're in a crisis, it's not that giving is good or giving is bad. You have to say, "During this hard time, what makes me feel better? What makes me feel worse?" It's not like there's a rule that when you're having a crisis you have to stop helping. You know, I take calls from friends of friends who have breast cancer and help them sort through their options. People say, "Oh, you do too much for people you don't even know," or "You're a saint," but it really doesn't take that much energy or time to help someone a whole lot, and it makes me feel really good. So taking those calls would not be on the list of things I would give up in a crisis. But if my daughter was still little and I was in a crisis, I would definitely give up driving car-pool! The message is not that you should change who you are in a crisis, but that you should figure out what is energizing to you and what isn't.

ALI: I agree!

Relationship Challenge: What to Do About a Broken Friendship

ALI: Sometimes we lose friends and we really miss them and want them back in our lives. But it's also possible to mature and then discover that a friend is just not healthy for you anymore, or to find that a friend makes a decision that is completely incompatible with your belief system. It's perfectly natural to outgrow friend-ships, and in fact it can be healthy to have a fight with a friend that ends things with a clean break. So first, you have to decide if a broken friendship is really worth mending.

SUSAN: Right now I'm thinking of one friend I lost—a cousin, ac-tually. We had lived in Boston at the same time and were really close. But when I came out, she stopped speaking to me. I missed her, so I kept sending Christmas cards to her and stuff like that, even though I got no response. Then, about ten years after she stopped talking to me, she went to the hospital for an emergency hysterectomy. She was so scared that she told all the doctors I was her cousin, because she hoped that having a connection in the medical world would get her better care. Afterward, she realized that she had basically rejected me but then expected me to do a favor for her in my absence! So she wrote me a long letter explaining all this and apologizing. I was glad to get it, and we became close again. Several years later, she died of cancer, and I was thankful we had reunited before it was too late.

ALI: That's interesting, because first your cousin did something awful, but then she grew and realized she had made a mistake. That happens. Sometimes it goes both ways. I had a stupid fight with a close friend, we stopped talking, and then a few years later another friend of mine died. So I bought a card that talked about the importance of friendship and wrote to the woman I'd fought with "Life is too short. I miss you. Can we be friends again?" I didn't hear from her for a few months, so I assumed she wasn't interested. But then she sent me a birthday card and asked me to call her, so we talked and now we're good friends again. A good give-and-take friendship can often be resurrected.

SUSAN: You can also reevaluate your expectations of a relationship, not just with friends but also with family members. Maybe, when your friend or sibling does something that annoys you, you'll have to say, "Oh well, that's just Susan!" And if you've been expecting too much, maybe *you're* the one who is the source of the rift.

ALI: If you've been a jerk, you have to own up to it. Apologize.

SUSAN: Most of the time, the other person will be happy to hear that you're back. You don't even have to offer a lot of excuses. In some cases, you can say, "I was in a different place back then, and I apologize, and I want our friendship back."

ALI: It doesn't take much to own up to a mistake and apologize sincerely.

SUSAN: Some people just can't, though. They can say, "I'm sorry you feel bad," not, "I'm sorry I did this stupid thing." You can understand friends like that and still love them.

ALI: Dave and I have this ongoing joke in which after a fight, the person whose fault it is has to take a specific amount of ownership for it. No fight is ever 100 percent the fault of just one person, so I might say, "I take ninety-three percent ownership of this fight," and Dave will say, "No, you should take ninety-four percent!" And sometimes he will say that this felt like a mutually stupid fight, and we should each take 50 percent blame and I will counter that, in fact, he should take 51 percent instead. And we usually end up laughing.

I think that if you really want to heal a friendship it's always worth trying. Sending a letter is a good idea because it's much easier to express complicated feelings in writing. It doesn't have to be long or eloquent. It can say something like, "I miss our friendship and I think of you often. I'm not even sure why we're not friends anymore, but I miss you."

Once, in high school, a group of close friends stopped talking to me. Many years later, one of them wrote to me and said, "We're sorry that we treated you so badly." I wrote back, "That's okay, but can you tell me what I did to make everyone so mad?" And she never wrote back. I still don't know what I did. It still bothers me a bit.

Caregiving: How Not to Drown

What about personal relationships in which you are a caregiver? Caregiving, whether it's raising a child or tending to a sick partner or an elderly parent, falls to many of us. By definition, this is an imbalanced relationship. The caregiver gives, and the recipient takes. Because we are often caring for people we love, our natural inclination as caregivers is to create an even bigger imbalance; we give, and give, and give some more. A study at the University of California at San Francisco compared mothers of healthy children with mothers of chronically disabled children, looking specifically at the women's telomeres (a sequence at the end of our chromosomes that becomes shorter with each cell division and is therefore a good marker of aging). Although the study was controlled for age, the mothers of disabled children—the mothers who tended to have many more caregiving duties—had telomeres that were, on average, between nine and fifteen years shorter. They were experiencing accelerated aging.

This study reveals some of the biology of what we already know: Spend too much time caring for others while neglecting yourself and you'll get sick—or maybe just irritable, resentful, and exhausted. If a true crisis arises with your loved one when you are already in this depleted state, how will you handle it?

The good news from this study is that there was a healthy subgroup of caregiving mothers, ones who had normal telomeres. These women also reported less stress from their duties than the other women did. The researchers concluded that it's not caregiving itself that makes you sick or stressed; it's how you perceive its burdens. If you can find a way to both provide good care and keep your stress under control, you're going to be okay.

What's the secret of women who give care without suffering excess stress? Accepting help and having social support. If someone offers to help, the highly adaptive caregivers don't say, "Thanks, but I've got it covered." They say, "You're the best! If I make you a list, can you pick up a few things at the grocery store for me this week?"

They also reach out for emotional assistance and sympathy. A lot of them join support groups. These groups can help reduce the pressure, because you realize that you're not alone in sometimes feeling resentful, or that you're not the only caregiver who has put on weight because there's no time to exercise. Even if you don't join a formal group, it helps to belong to a casual network of people who are in the same boat. Last year, Ali was at one of her kids' softball games when she looked down at the sandwiches she'd packed, and groaned. She said to the parents around her, "My kids have had so many sports events this month that we've had sandwiches for dinner *thirteen nights* in a row." For a minute she felt like a marginally inadequate mom because her family had eaten only one home-cooked meal in the last two weeks. But then all the other parents laughed sympathetically and chimed in with comments like, "That's nothing. We've been eating cereal every night for a month!"

If you can talk to people who are in positions similar to yours, you realize that successful caregivers—and this includes parents—don't even try to do it all. They don't serve piping hot dinners, they don't have immaculate homes, and they definitely don't clean the crumbs out from under the toaster. They understand that they can choose: They can chase perfection in every detail of their lives, or they can be happy. Above all, they realize that superwomen don't fly. They drown.

Relationship Challenge: When You're a Caregiver of Elderly Parents and Need More Help from Your Siblings

ALI: You should think about this in the same way you should think about managing stress, in terms of needs and resources. What are your parents' needs, and what are the resources available? Figure out what your parents need that they are unable to supply on their own. Include physical needs (maybe someone to lift them into the bathtub) but also what they require emotionally, financially, intellectually, and socially. Then list the resources you have on hand for meeting those needs. And then list the resources your sibs have.

SUSAN: But that might not be fair. Maybe the reason your sibling isn't helping is that she's just not able to do it right now.

ALI: That's the point of this exercise. It clarifies what your siblings can and can't do. It's fair to be angry with a sibling who refuses to help with the caregiving in any way, but it's not fair to be angry with a sibling who lives on the other side of the continent and can't do a lot of the physical labor. So then you sit down with siblings or call them, and look at your lists. Who has more time? Maybe that person can do more of the physical caregiving. Who has energy? That sibling can make all the phone calls to doctors' offices and insurance companies. Who has money? That sibling can pay for home health care or even a nursing home.

SUSAN: Or a sibling who can't or won't come out to help can do Internet research. He or she can find out what caregiving services are available. Meals on Wheels, maybe, or adult day care, or respite care for you.

ALI: When my mother was ill, my sister and I split the tasks according to what each of us was good at. What you *don't* want is for the impatient, businesslike sib to make all the phone calls to your parents' friends or speak with the church or synagogue. The job for that sib is to talk to the insurance companies! When you look at your resources, you can come up with a plan that's more likely to work, because your siblings can help by doing what they're best at.

SUSAN: Sometimes there are siblings who just can't do much at all.

ALI: It sounds harsh, but if your sibs are unwilling or unable to help, you need to be clear that if your parents have financial resources, you are going to draw on some of that money to help pay for caregiving. When you say this, often you will find that siblings who were too busy are suddenly available to help out.

SUSAN: I'm worried that we're focusing too much on women who are taking care of their parents. There are so many women with disabled or sick kids. We can't leave them out.

ALI: This idea can apply to those women, too, but it's a little different because you may not be calling on siblings for help as much as from your whole family or your circle of friends. It's true that both scenarios are very hard. If you are taking care of a very elderly and sick parent, you know there is an end in sight. But if you are taking care of a disabled child, you may be a caregiver for a very long time. In this instance you really need support, because you've got to stay healthy for the long haul.

Healthy Sex Lives

We always get a good snicker out of television shows that claim to depict women's lives realistically. There are the obligatory whining kids, high-stress jobs, competitive neighbors, and difficult marriages or partnerships. But despite her crammed schedule, when it comes to sex this exhausted, stressed-out, "real" woman is invariably eager for more, more, more! (Wonder how many men are on the screenwriting teams for these shows?)

Of course, many women love sex, and lots of it. We just wish that the entire spectrum of sexual appetites could be acknowledged as "real," from the voracious to the please-just-let-me-sleep varieties. It's totally normal, even common, for a woman to want sex most days of the week. It's also normal to have a much lower libido; many women want sex less frequently. Over a lifetime, a woman's desire may wax and wane according to hormones, caregiving duties, work pressures, and stress levels, as well as the ups and downs of long-term relationships. Or not. What *isn't* healthy is for you and your partner to constantly struggle over which one of you has the "normal" sex drive, and which is a sex maniac / Frigidaire.

From now on, feel free to ignore any "expert" who proclaims you need to have sex X number of times per week or month, and instead focus on the real questions: Are you comfortable with your sex life? Are you having much more or much less sex than you want to? And if you and your partner aren't well matched in terms of sexual appetites, can you compromise on frequency without feeling either deprived or submissive?

In her work with couples, Ali has found that people are often not as far apart in their desires as it seems. It's just that people who want more sex are afraid that if they don't ask for it every day, they'll *never* get it. By the same token, people who want less sex are afraid that if they say yes too often, their partners will never learn to restrain themselves. And so they end up with one partner constantly asking for sex and the other constantly refusing. Note that we are not saying that men are always asking for sex and women are always refusing. There are many couples where the wife wishes their frequency would increase and the husband is not that interested. Don't assume that men always want more sex than women, because the opposite is common as well.

The solution is to bring the subject out into the light and ask, "How often would you like to have sex?" Often the "sex maniac" wants sex, say, three times a week and the "Frigidaire" wants it once, on the weekend. For a couple with a basically healthy relationship, that's hardly an irreconcilable difference. When couples really do have radically different sex drives—every day versus once a month or even once a year—it may be time for therapy. A good therapist can guide a couple through this and work toward helping each partner feel happy with his or her sex life. Sometimes it is a matter of reassuring one or both partners that masturbation is truly healthy and acceptable, sometimes it comes down to educating each partner about how to satisfy the other, and sometimes one or both issues need to be referred to a physician to rule out physical problems. There are many medical conditions and medications that can cause or contribute to an unusually low sex drive; appropriate treatment or a switch in medication can often resolve the issue.

Relationship Challenge: When You Need More Support from Your Partner with the Kids or the Chores

ALI: What I do with my patients—and I see this problem a *lot* in my practice—is to have them spend a week noticing everything that needs doing in their home and life and write it down. This includes stuff with the kids, shopping, errands, cleaning, buying birthday presents . . . you should jot down everything. Then look at how much really needs to get done. Try to come up with a list of reasonable basics. You don't need to scrub the baseboards with a toothbrush every week, but you do need to eat and have clean clothes. Then divvy up the items, but don't just go down the list and say, "I get item number one, you get item number two, I get number three." Divide the tasks according to your strengths. If mowing the lawn is on the list and he's better at it than you are and doesn't mind doing it, *he* should be doing it. I don't mind washing dishes, but I hate taking out the garbage, so Dave does that and I wash the dishes. And if there are chores that both of you hate, divide them up equally.

SUSAN: Or hire somebody! And if you're the one who can't stand to do the work, then *you're* the one who has to do the hiring.

ALI: Paying somebody to come clean the house or mow the lawn can be cheaper than paying a couples counselor!

SUSAN: Well, you might have a partner who refuses to divide up the tasks or even to sit down with a list.

ALI: Then you're back to the same options. If your partner won't split the work, say that you'll hire someone to do the work or you have to go into couples counseling. But you have to be fair. Your partner might do more than you realize. I knew a woman who was a partner in a big law firm, and she spent a lot of time being angry with her stay-at-home husband for not doing enough around the house. Then she quit and he got a job—and she realized just how much there was to do every day. On the other hand, if your husband is gone all day and you're at home, it's not fair to expect him to come straight home from work and make dinner for all of you.

SUSAN: I don't know about that last one. You have to be careful about assuming that the person who is at home has an easier life than the person who works. When my daughter was four, I worked full-time as a surgeon. And it was my responsibility to get her dressed and then drive her to preschool. I used to say that the hour with Katie was the hardest part of my day; the rest of it was only life and death! Because I had control over surgery. When I asked for a clamp, I got one. Nobody said "Why? *Why?* WHY?"

the way Katie did when it was time to put on her shoes. If the two of you have been evenly splitting the chores, and then one of you gets a big promotion or one of you stays home with the children, negotiating that shift can be difficult.

ALI: When there's a shift, you have to be fluid for a while. In theory, you and your partner may be committed to sharing child care duties. But if your partner is working full-time and you're home with the baby, does it make sense to ask your partner to wake up for midnight feedings? You can always nap during the day, but your partner can't.

SUSAN: It doesn't always work out that way. We just had some friends stay with us who have a toddler and a newborn, and, boy, that's tough. The father, who stays home, is completely exhausted by the time his wife gets home from work. It's different in all relationships. You have to negotiate things according to your own situation and your partner's.

ALI: Okay, but make the list.

SUSAN: Oh, yeah! Make the list.

Uh . . . *Duh!*

According to the *New York Times,* the unhappiest people in America are the ones who live with teenagers.

Quiz: Are Your Relationships Pretty Healthy?

When it comes to social support, sex, and caregiving, do you give, give, give? Or take, take, take? Hopefully, you do some of both. To determine whether your relationships are in the Pretty Healthy Zone for social support, answer the questions below. Circle your answers, then add up your points and read about your score.

1. Close friends are people in whom you can confide your worries, troubles, and joys. How many people in your life meet that definition? Family members count.

0 points. There is no one I trust enough to confide in.

1 point. I have a couple of friends I can really talk to.

2 points. I have four or five close friends, plus a handful of others who can be there for me in a pinch.

3 points. I'm an open book. Anyone who knows me also knows my whole life story.

2. Is there a balance between how much you give to your relationships and how much support you receive in return?

0 points. I don't have anyone in my life, so when it comes to giving and taking, there's not much of either.

1 point. I've got a lot going on, so I tend to ask more from people than I can give back.

2 points. If I look back over the past few years, I've had times of giving and of taking. I'm there for my friends in times of crises, and they are there for me.

3 points. I'm the one my friends can count on whenever they need somebody, but when times are tough for me, I can handle it all on my own.

(continued)

3. Are there people currently in your life who have actually helped you out when you needed them?

0 points. No, none.

1 point. There are a couple of people who have helped me out before, but when I get into a jam I often notice that I could use more support.

2 points. Time and again, my friends have proven their willingness to help me.

3 points. Sometimes I wonder if I have too much support. My friends are overinvolved in my life, giving me advice and encouraging me to talk about my problems even when I want to keep things private.

4. Do you have sex as often as you'd like?

0 points. I'm not having sex at all these days, but not because I don't want to.

1 point. Sometimes I'm irritated when my partner initiates sex, but once things get going I'm happy to participate.

2 points. My sex drive has changed over the years, but in general, the frequency of sex has matched my needs.

3 points. I have sex way more often than I'd like because I want to keep my partner happy.

5. Which of the following best describes the quality of your orgasms?

0 points. Orgasm? What's an orgasm?

1 point. It's hit or miss. If I'm not in exactly the right mood, it doesn't happen for me.

2 points. Most of the time I achieve orgasm, and I'm satisfied with that.

(continued)

3 points. I'm capable of multiple orgasms, which sounds great—but it means that I'm frustrated if I have only one.

6. Describe the level of intimacy in your romantic relationship.

0 points. I'm starving. I crave the emotional and physical intimacy that I lack.

1 point. I don't have a romantic partner, but I don't feel like I'm missing a whole lot.

2 points. Most of the time I feel a satisfying level of sensuality and intimacy with my partner.

3 points. I could use a little more space. Sometimes we're so intimate that I feel overpowered.

7. How much caregiving do you perform?

0 points. I don't see myself as the caregiving type. When people need me, I tend to do the minimum—or I hire someone to do the job—and then escape to freedom.

1 point. I have no responsibility for anyone, although I'd like to contribute to someone else's life.

2 points. Caregiving is one aspect of my vibrant, full life. I am sometimes busier than I'd like to be, but overall my caregiving responsibilities are manageable.

3 points. I am so busy with caregiving duties that there is no time left in my life for anything else.

8. How much support do you get for your caregiving duties?

0 points. I refuse to take on any caregiving responsibilities, so I don't need support in that area.

(continued)

1 point. I don't get or need much help on a daily or weekly basis, but there are people who will come to my aid if I have a serious caregiving crisis.

2 points. My friends and family help me with my caregiving duties whenever I ask.

3 points. I've asked and asked, but no one is willing to lighten my caregiving load.

9. How comfortable do you feel asking for help from friends and/or family members? (This can include, but is not limited to, help with caregiving.)

0 points. This question doesn't apply to me. I take pride in handling my own problems.

1 point. I'm so good at delegating that there's not much left for *me* to do. Now that I think about it, my friends and family have seemed kind of irritated with me lately.

2 points. I've become pretty good at calling friends and asking for what I need, though I try not to take advantage of them.

3 points. I gratefully receive help from my friends, but asking for a specific favor is tough for me. Sometimes I end up with dozens of casseroles in my freezer when what I really need is someone to drive my mother to get her lab work done.

Scoring

0–9 points: You seem to be isolated, which is a cause for concern. Check in with your doctor to make sure that depression is not a cause or a result of being alone. Then make an effort to build more ties; if you don't have family or friends nearby, volunteer work can be a good place to start. You can also see page 67 for ways to meet people whose company you might enjoy.

(continued)

10–15 points: You're not lonely, and you're not socially overwhelmed, which earns you a spot in the PH Zone. There may be times when you long for greater human connection; this may mean that you need to give as much to your relationships as you'd like to get out of them.

15–21 points: Your friends and family keep you busy, but overall you have quality relationships with a satisfying element of give-and-take. Your relationships are definitely Pretty Healthy.

22–27 points: You have passed through the PH Zone for relationships . . . and landed on the other side. You need to examine the relationships in your life and figure out how to keep those that are healthy and satisfying while changing those that are depleting you. If you are a caregiver, make it a priority to get more support for your work.

Chapter Eight

A Pretty Healthy Life, Decade by Decade

YOU DON'T NEED US TO tell you that women's bodies are constantly changing—from girlhood to puberty to young adulthood; from motherhood to menopause and beyond. Our health needs change, too. Any forty-five-year-old woman, whose body is surfing a new wave of hormones practically every day, is aware of this simple fact. Yet a lot of the health "noise" that blasts out of our computers, televisions, magazines, and newspapers is focused on diseases and disorders that tend to strike most forcefully at elderly women, not the general female population. As a result, we worry too much about illnesses that may be very far off and are blind to present health threats. That's why women in their twenties are terrified if they forget to perform a monthly breast self-exam but fail to protect themselves against sexually transmitted diseases.

To give you a more realistic look at health across different ages, we present "A Pretty Healthy Life," a decade-by-decade analysis of women's risks and challenges. You'll see a timeline that presents the top causes of death for each age bracket. Although it's never pleasant to think about dying, we find this timeline strangely calming. It discredits the idea that heart disease and cancer are lurking around every corner, at every stage of life.

We'll also go through the decades, starting with the twenties and ending with the seventies and eighties, presenting our guidelines for pretty good health and discussing how to handle the health obstacles that arise as women pass in and out of childbearing, career building, caregiving, hot flashing, retiring, and grandparenting. Each decade also brings with it pleasant surprises and opportunities. If you're not going to relax and enjoy the triple-fudge brownies when you're eighty-five, then when?

Twenties

A GENERATION AGO, elders struggled to convince the younger crowd that life does not, in fact, last forever. ("You kids think you're immortal! You'll see!") These days, few young women need this kind of warning. Thanks to the steady thrum of medical warnings, they are constantly confronted with their mortality:

The leading cause of death in women is heart disease.

Your odds of contracting breast cancer are 1 in 8.

And so they start to fear diseases that are statistically unlikely to occur until they are much older. We think it's sad to see beautiful young women who've been taught to think of their hearts and breasts as ticking time bombs, at an age when they should be enjoying their bodies.

The facts are your best weapon against fear mongering. Although heart disease is the number one cause of death for women, most of those deaths occur in women in their seventies and beyond. Yes, some young women have heart attacks, but it happens only rarely—and the vast majority of these cases are caused by congenital abnormalities, not lifestyle choices, meaning that their heart attacks were not caused by infrequent exercise or too much pizza. The same goes for strokes. And the odds of developing breast cancer at age twenty-five are 1 in 20,000. Most other cancer rates are also low at this age. If you are in your twenties, you definitely don't need mammograms (no, not even "just to be extra sure"), and, as we have explained before, you don't need to perform formal breast self-exams at any age.

The two of us debated the importance of traditional health habits—eating well, exercise, stress management—for twenty-something women, and here's how the conversation went:

ALI: You can get away with more in your twenties, when poor diet, lack of exercise, and lack of sleep won't have quite the same health implications as later in life. Nevertheless, it's best to set up those habits when you're young. Lock them down now, and the rest of your life will be *much* easier.

SUSAN: That's too restrictive! Women in their twenties have a lot on their plates. They're sweating out entry-level jobs that don't pay very well. There's the indignity of being low woman on the totem pole and having a boss who may come down hard on you, which is especially tough for girls who grew up in the Age of Affirmation . . . you know, they received cheers and a trophy for everything they did, including sitting on the bench of the losing soccer team. And they're trying to figure out who they are. It's a good idea for twenty-somethings to exercise to relieve stress,

Risk Chart For Women

Find the line closest to your age and smoking status.¹ The numbers tell you **how many of 1,000 women will die in the next ten years from . . .**

Age	Smoking	VASCULAR DISEASE		CANCER					INFECTION			LUNG DISEASE	ACCIDENTS	ALL CAUSES COMBINED*
		Heart Disease	Stroke	Lung	Breast	Colon	Ovarian	Cervical	Pneumonia	Flu	AIDS	COPD		
35	Never smoker	1	1		1						1		2	14
	Smoker	**1**	**1**	**1**	**1**						**1**		**2**	**14**
40	Never smoker	1			2	1					1		2	19
	Smoker	**4**	**2**	**4**	**2**						**1**	**1**	**2**	**27**
45	Never smoker	2	1	1	3	1	1				1		2	25
	Smoker	**9**	**3**	**7**	**3**	**1**	**1**		**1**		**1**	**2**	**2**	**45**
50	Never smoker	4	1	1	4	1	1						2	37
	Smoker	**13**	**5**	**14**	**4**	**1**	**1**		**1**			**4**	**2**	**69**

Fewer than 1 death

Age													
55	Never smoker	8	2	2	6	2	2	1	1		1	2	55
	Smoker	**20**	**6**	**26**	**5**	**2**	**2**	**1**	**1**		**9**	**2**	**110**
60	Never smoker	14	4	3	7	3	3	1	1		2	2	84
	Smoker	**31**	**8**	**41**	**6**	**3**	**3**	**1**	**2**		**18**	**2**	**167**
65	Never smoker	25	7	5	8	4	4	1	2		3	3	131
	Smoker	**45**	**15**	**55**	**7**	**3**	**3**	**1**	**4**		**31**	**3**	**241**
70	Never smoker	46	14	7	9	4	4	1	4		5	4	207
	Smoker	**66**	**25**	**61**	**8**	**4**	**4**	**1**	**7**		**44**	**4**	**335**
75	Never smoker	86	30	7	10	5	5	1	8		6	7	335
	Smoker	**99**	**34**	**58**	**10**	**9**	**4**		**14**		**61**	**7**	**463**

ªA never smoker has smoked fewer than one hundred cigarettes in her life, and a current smoker has smoked at least one hundred cigarettes or more in her life and smokes (any amount) now.

*The numbers in each row do not add up to the chance of dying from everything combined, because there are many other causes of death besides the ones listed here.

and they shouldn't put on too much weight because it's so hard to take off later, but don't tell them they have to figure out their health habits for the rest of their lives. It's not like it's now or never.

ALI: But think about a young woman who is just out of school or college and starting to work. In college, she probably had twenty-four-hour access to a multimillion-dollar exercise facility. Now she'll have to pay a lot of money if she wants to join a gym, or she'll have to wake up early if she decides to go running before work. She used to have a pediatrician who gave her complete checkups, and then a student health center where she could drop in whenever she had a problem. Now she will have to make decisions about getting a primary care doctor and an ob-gyn, and she'll have to learn to advocate for her own health. On campus, there was always a salad bar available. Now she has to buy or make her own food. And if she developed flagrantly bad habits earlier, like smoking or drinking too much, isn't now a good time to stop?

SUSAN: I see what you mean, especially in that last point. A lot of women start to drink or do drugs or smoke in their twenties. If you already have one or more of these habits, this could be a great age for making big changes, maybe by hanging out with a different group of friends. And if you're not overwhelmed by work or grad school, you could try answering some of those other health questions. But don't feel bad if you just can't figure them all out. You're not doomed to a lifetime of bad health if you don't. You have plenty of time left.

Although it's great if you can establish good eating and exercising habits in your twenties, we think it's even more important for you to consider your safety. Now it's our turn to sound the alarm, although we're doing so with the statistics to back us up: The true leading cause of death for women in their twenties is unintentional accidents—car crashes, diving into shallow water, falls, and other events none of us likes to think about. To be Pretty Healthy in your twenties, you don't need to shy away from adventure; just protect yourself by taking the obvious, standard, boring measures:

- Wear your seat belt.
- Don't drink more than you should.
- Don't drive under the influence or get into a car with an impaired driver.
- Wear a helmet when you ride a bike or participate in any other sport that could result in head injury.

Of course, you can't completely dismiss all other health concerns in your twenties. You'll hate to hear this, but your high school sex-ed teacher was right: Sexually transmitted diseases are real. Not just HIV and AIDS, but also extremely unpleasant STDs like chlamydia, gonorrhea, and herpes. Practice safe sex and use a condom, even if you are on the Pill.

Finally, it's a good idea to keep your fertility in mind. Your ability to conceive peaks at around age twenty-five, and although it's not politically correct to say so, the younger you are when you have children, the lower your risk of breast cancer. Please don't rush out and get pregnant out of fear that *when you turn thirty your ovaries will shrivel up like raisins* (they won't), but if you feel ready for kids and have all the ingredients in place to support them, maybe you'll want to buck the trend and try to get pregnant sooner rather than later.

How to Be Pretty Healthy in Your Twenties

- Protect yourself against accidents and injury (see page 199).
- Practice safe sex.
- Get the cervical cancer vaccine by age twenty-six.
- Take stock of your stress levels. Do you have ways to relieve stress? If not, try some of the techniques in chapter 3.
- Ask your parents or other relatives about your family's health history, both physical and mental. Record this information so that you and your physician can refer to it in the coming years.
- Figure out how you will get adequate health insurance.
- Get annual Pap tests until you have had two or three negative results in a row; after that, you can go three years between Paps. If you are sexually active, get regular screenings for STDs.
- Break any seriously bad health habits, like smoking, binge eating, substance abuse, or drinking to excess. You might need some professional support here, but the extra cost and time will be well worth it.
- Start thinking about your fertility; you don't need to get pregnant right now, but it's nice to avoid the "I forgot to get pregnant!" syndrome in your forties.
- Try to set up good patterns of eating, sleeping, and exercising well, but *not out of fear.* Getting rid of bad habits is more important at this age than becoming obsessed with health perfection.

Thirties

BETTE MIDLER ONCE said that you know you're a grown-up when you finally go out and buy a bath mat. It's in our thirties that most of us start to feel like card-carrying (and bath-mat-buying) adults.

You still need to follow the childhood motto of "Safety first," however. Wear seat belts in the car, protective gear when playing sports, and drink moderately. Sexually transmitted diseases remain a danger, so keep practicing safe sex. *"I've always been lucky"* is not a Pretty Healthy approach to sexual health.

The good news is that heart disease, cancer, and other major disablers are still unlikely to happen to you. There are always exceptions, especially if you have a strong family history of certain diseases, but for most of you these health problems should not be your primary concern. What really changes in your thirties is your level of stress. Yes, your twenties were a time of growth, which was definitely stressful. But now stress flies at you from all angles—career, kids, home, parents—and it can hit hard.

At work, things are both better and worse than they were in your twenties. You're probably not fetching coffee and making copies anymore. You have more independence; you're tougher; you're exercising more of your powers. But there are some people who wish you had stayed a sweet young thing. Growing up means you also have to learn to deal effectively with people who've come to see you as a threat. (Start by choosing to view their competitive behavior as a compliment.)

For some women, infertility is a major struggle during this decade. There are plenty of women in their thirties who have trouble getting pregnant. If you are age thirty-five or under and have been trying for a year without success, it is time to see an infertility specialist. If you are between ages thirty-five and forty, wait only six months. The sooner you seek help, the more likely you are to get pregnant. And contrary to what you may hear, the majority of women who get treatment are able to have a healthy baby, often by using simple and noninvasive approaches. But don't let anyone tell you otherwise: Being infertile in a fertile world is extremely stressful.

If you have kids, your thirties tend to be dominated by the sleep-deprived consumption of leftover sandwich crusts. Sleep deprivation is stressful all by itself, and it can be made worse if you believe you will suffer lasting physical or mental damage as a result. You won't. We don't want you to become so worn down that you are a mere little nubbin of your former lively self, so try to get rest when you can. But during those tough nights when you are walking the floors with a sick child, you can hold on to our promise that you will live to sleep again (until menopause, at least, when sleeplessness makes a comeback). And about those sandwich crusts: It's certainly okay to let things go for a little while—especially while your baby is brand-new—but remember that weight is much easier to put on than to take off. We know a woman who gained seventy-five pounds just by finishing off her kids' ants on a log (you know, celery stuffed with peanut butter and topped with raisins) and leftover mac and cheese. You don't want to enter your forties with a lot of extra weight if you can help it, because then your metabolism slows and it's even tougher to lose the pounds.

But don't let sleep deprivation and weight gain distract you from other sources of new-family stress. A lot of women put their careers on hold, which can generate an identity crisis if you previously defined yourself by your job title. You and your spouse are probably suffering a difficult transition as you negotiate a whole new set of responsibilities and roles, especially if you have bought a home to raise those kiddies in. ("Get up with the baby at night? Why should *I* get up with the baby? *I* pay the mortgage *on this house!*")

For all these reasons and more (you can probably think of a few yourself), stress management should become one of your top health priorities in your thirties. Try out several stress-relieving strategies until you find a few that suit you best (several are listed in chapter 3), and use them often. Take time every day, even if it's just a few minutes, to practice self-care. For Ali, this means winding down at night by reading the newspaper. Susan likes to practice the piano (when she is not busy rear-ending cars on the freeway, that is).

Finally, learn the warning signs of stress overload: headaches, gastrointestinal symptoms, fatigue, insomnia, irritability, increased alcohol intake, and cravings for junk food. And whatever help you need, get it or take it.

How to Be Pretty Healthy in Your Thirties

- Protect yourself against accidents and injury (see page 199).
- Practice safe sex.
- Learn stress management techniques and use them.
- Get help if you experience the symptoms of stress overload.
- If you've been going in for annual Pap tests and have had two or three negative results in a row, you can start waiting three years between tests. Continue screening for STDs.
- If you'd like to have children but haven't started a family yet, continue to keep your fertility in mind.
- Try to avoid responding to stress by overeating or engaging in other unhealthy behaviors.
- Don't panic about garden-variety sleep loss, but do listen to your body. If you are exhausted, error-prone, and falling apart, something needs to change.
- If you don't exercise regularly, start thinking about it more seriously. At this age, chances are that you are naturally fit enough to avoid the worst consequences of inactivity—but be aware that exercise can improve your mood as well as your sleep.

- Eat good foods, but don't be discouraged if you eat poorly during the occasional crisis. Return to eating wholesome foods once life goes back to normal.

Forties

IN YOUR TWENTIES and thirties, you could probably pass some basic fitness measures (such as running a mile without stopping; see pages 111–13), even if you never worked out. Now that you're forty, there's no escaping it: *You've got to get yourself in gear.* In this decade, you start to lose a lot of the natural fitness you had in your youth. Your daily activity also tends to slow down, perhaps because you no longer live in an urban downtown where you can walk to work, or because you're not getting your natural strength training by lifting small children. A more formal exercise program can help you maintain your strength and energy. And not to spook you, but in your forties, your risk of heart disease and cancer leaps out of the "probably negligible" territory and into the category of "this might happen to *me*!" But it appears that fit people are less vulnerable to these diseases. The good news is that you may have more time to work out, now that you're past the crazy-busy thirties.

Or maybe not. For some women, the forties are a time to enjoy a mature self-knowledge. If they have families, their kids are probably in school full-time and they can breathe (and sleep) once again. But other women are devoting themselves to dealing with infertility, because it's so hard to achieve a spontaneous, healthy pregnancy after the age of forty-three. Women who have babies in their late thirties or early forties may find themselves in the double bind of raising young children while caring for ailing parents. In this circumstance it's enormously difficult—but still necessary—to put self-care on your to-do list.

Contrary to popular belief, menopause is defined as the point at which you have not had a period for a full year. But the symptoms of menopause are actually at their most severe in the years leading up to it. This time is called perimenopause, and you might notice its first symptoms in your mid- to late forties. Susan likes to describe perimenopause as puberty in reverse. Like puberty, perimenopause consists of about three or four years when you're gearing up for a major hormonal adjustment. Your hormone levels ratchet themselves up, plummet downward, and then spike again in unpredictable bursts. You can feel bitchy and bloated and pimply, and your brain doesn't work the way it's supposed to. You have hot flashes, although these often aren't as bad as most women fear. And then, eventually, your hormones even themselves out and you reach a "new normal." The major difference between puberty and menopause is that now you are wiser and more capable. You can cruise through these shifts with more aplomb. And at the end, you won't have periods anymore! Imagine: You can pack for vacation and not have to ask yourself: Will I need paper products on this trip? Use the extra space in your suitcase for a great book or some fizzy bath confection.

We think that the real challenge of your forties is not perimenopause but another natural process: midlife assessment. Years ago, doctors were taught that women in their forties suffered from depression caused by decreased estrogen levels, but most of the studies behind this theory were poorly conducted. Now we know that *both* men and women struggle with depression in their forties, especially their late forties. At this age, it's hard not to compare your childhood fantasy of adult life to the life you lead now—and, understandably, comparing fantasy to reality is a deflating experience. Get help if you feel depressed—and take heart. This reassessment is painful, but it gives you the opportunity to build a solid foundation for the next forty or fifty years.

Weight gain seems to creep up on women by their mid-forties, but this is not such a bad thing. An increase of five to ten pounds (but no more than that) may be biologically desirable. Why? For one thing, it looks as if being somewhat plump can lead to a longer life, and the extra weight is also natural bone protection. If you slip and fall when you are older, a little natural padding—especially on your hips—can cushion the blow. In fact, low weight (not low bone density) is the number one predictor of debilitating falls in old age. So if you gain weight and are upset by it, ask yourself: *Would I rather gain ten pounds now, or wear hip pads when I'm seventy?* Until we get the word that Marc Jacobs is planning a new line of couture hip pads, we'll take the pounds.

How to Be Pretty Healthy in Your Forties

- Exercise (this includes strength training).
- Eat good foods, but know that it's normal to gain between five and ten pounds during this decade.
- Take time to nurture yourself, especially if you are sandwiched between caring for a younger generation and an older one.
- Take the symptoms of perimenopause in stride; you are merely going through puberty in reverse.
- Remember that it's possible to get pregnant during perimenopause. Use contraception until it's been one full year since your last period. (Even then, you still need to practice safe sex.)
- Know the symptoms of depression, and get help if you need it.

Fifties

HERE IS THE one-sentence story of your fifties: You go through menopause, and then things get better.

If you did not begin perimenopause in your forties, then you will in your fifties. After you've had one full year without periods, menopause is officially over. Your hormones even out. Your moods will be steadier, your complexion will improve, and sleep will return (well, probably). Now is a great time to think of all those hot flashes as power surges. How will you use *your* new power? To go back to school, back to work, grow a business? You may still have older children or ailing parents to watch over, and you're probably not ready for retirement. But you can start asking yourself some provocative questions.

Just as you start to imagine your prospects in vivid detail, you may come up hard against hints of your mortality. You can't read without your glasses. You're creaky at the knees. It's harder to hear in crowds. You say, "Let's eat out early because I don't sleep so well when I have a big meal . . . and I'm planning to be in bed by nine-thirty." You may find yourself on medication for high blood pressure, or you may even develop a chronic disease. But you're still yourself, and your body is still your friend. Even if you have limitations you have enough wisdom now to compensate for them.

In your fifties, heart disease and cancer take on a new reality. It is likely that someone you know—and someone who is your age—will die from one of these causes. It is hard not to think: *What did my friend do wrong to die so young? What can I do differently?* The trick is to understand that no one has total control over her health—and then exercise, eat wisely, and manage stress anyway. Susan recalls thinking when she turned fifty:

> *I would hate to die young because I didn't feel like exercising or eating good food. I would hate for my grandkids to miss out on knowing their full extended family because I was lazy. That's what gets me up for my morning runs. That, and the fact that I will feel better if I do. I want to be around with a good quality of life. But the flip side is that I could always get hit by a car! I can't control every single thing.*

Fortunately, it's easier to focus on good health habits than it was before. If you don't have ravenous kids around, you don't tend to buy as many graham crackers and quarts of ice cream—or to eat them. You can dash out of the house to exercise without consulting someone else's schedule or making sure there is someone at home to watch the kids. If you've never had kids, you'll find it easier to maintain your social network now that your peers aren't so preoccupied with their broods. At work, you probably have more control over your time than you used to, either because you've risen in the ranks, or simply because you've been around long enough to know how to work within the system.

In general, your fifties are a time of greater confidence and authority. Even if your financial or marital circumstances aren't great, you should have enough self-esteem to pick and choose how you spend your free time and with whom you spend it. At this marvelous age, you have both time and health. Use them.

How to Be Pretty Healthy in Your Fifties

- Exercise (this includes strength training).
- Eat good foods.

- Take the symptoms of perimenopause in stride; you are merely going through puberty in reverse.
- Remember that although it's not likely you will get pregnant in your fifties, it's possible. Use contraception until it's been one full year since your last period. (Even then, you still need to practice safe sex.)
- If you are not happy and content, it's time to figure out why.
- Continue with health screenings as needed. In particular, start getting mammograms every year or two, and schedule your first colonoscopy.

Sixties

IN YOUR SIXTIES, your body starts to show some signs of wear and tear, and you start to see a more direct connection between healthy habits and your sense of well-being. We women were built for long, arduous lives, so although we are less likely than men to contract swift, brutal diseases, we're more likely to develop chronic ailments, such as arthritis and high blood pressure. If you're going to live well, you will need the resilience that comes from regular physical activity and eating good foods. Your risk of serious problems, such as cancer, clogged arteries, and diabetes, grows as well, and most of us are willing to take the bet that clean, active living will reduce the risk of these diseases. But don't go overboard.

If you try to make yourself immortal by following a radically low-fat, low-salt, low-calorie, low-everything diet, within a few months you'll be so miserable you'll *wish* you could drop dead of a heart attack. (Maybe in heaven the food will be better.) Instead, make your philosophy "all things in moderation, including spaghetti carbonara."

It's both easier and harder to maintain good habits in your sixties. These are the tea-and-toast years, when your appetite may be less voracious—good news for women who have struggled with their weight for decades, but a challenge for those of you who need to put on some protective padding around your bones. Now you have more time for exercise . . . and you'll need it. No longer can you jump out of bed on a fine spring morning, and, after a winter of hibernating in front of the television, decide to ride twenty miles on your bike. In your sixties, you'll have to work up to new exercise routines more carefully, more gradually.

You may also have some limitations because of twitchy knees or creaky bones, in which case you'll have to reevaluate your ability to participate in certain sports. Expect to spend a while experimenting with the alternatives. If running or tennis starts to hurt a lot, would you like to try swimming? Walking? Cycling? Your workouts should now include some balance work as well as strength training.

You may find that, having survived your party days and your mothering years, sleep is once again hard to come by. It's not so difficult to fall asleep at this age, but staying asleep may be tough. (A cognitive-behavioral approach has been proven to improve sleep consolidation, so give it a try. See pages 30–33.) If this and other measures don't help, don't despair. Some sleep loss is normal as we get older, and if you generally feel good during the day, you probably aren't suffering major ill effects from your restless nights.

As important as exercise, eating well, and good sleep are, don't overlook another health topic: your relationships. Your bonds with other people are critically important to your well-being as you get older . . . which is just when some of those bonds are starting to weaken. If you have moved as a result of retirement; if your husband or partner is older and becoming disabled; or if your grown-up kids have become fully independent from you, then it's time to cast about for new sources of social support. Fortunately, by now you have a strong sense of yourself and may be more comfortable identifying potential new friends. Better still, you have been through several of life's ups and downs, and you've developed more hardiness.

Health screenings—which once involved nothing more than an occasional mini-checkup—take center stage in your sixties. You should continue to get mammograms every year or two, and you'll need your first bone density scan when you turn age sixty-five. Colonoscopies, blood work, and other tests are necessary, too (see pages 93–95 for a very basic list) and may vary according to your personal and family health history. One of your challenges now is to avoid seeing yourself as a walking bundle of risk factors. ("I'm high LDL cholesterol, with a family history of diabetes. In other words, I'm done for!") Remember that a risk factor can help you and your doctor think about your needs, but it's not the same as fate.

Try to control what you can with lifestyle measures and possibly medications . . . and then let go of the things you can't control. For example, being sixty-five drastically increases the odds that your body will not look the way it did when you were twenty. So let that fantasy go! It's *wonderful* when you no longer feel the pressure to wear high heels or keep your roots touched up.

Your sixties are the sweet spot of life, that lovely time between the hard work of growing up and the slower years of old age. If you were driven by ambition in your younger years, now you can explore new friendships and passions. If you stayed at home to raise a family, you might be ready to go back to school or back to business. It's no coincidence that the women who've made the biggest splashes in the world have been postmenopausal: Golda Meir, Margaret Thatcher, Hillary Clinton, Barbara Boxer, and loads of other heroines who see their children into independence and then come in to their own.

How to Be Pretty Healthy in Your Sixties

- Exercise (this includes strength training as well as balance work).
- Eat good foods. If you are already slender, be wary of losing any more weight.
- If you have trouble sleeping, try the suggestions listed in chapter 2.
- Work on maintaining old relationships and forging new ones.
- Wear your seat belt and other protective gear as necessary, because you can still have accidents.
- Get your first bone density screening at age sixty-five and remember to continue your mammograms. Other health screenings are important, too (see pages 93–95).
- Practice safe sex.
- Create a living will. Clearly describe your wishes to the people who are closest to you.
- Remember that health habits are supposed to help you enjoy life, not make it miserable!

Seventies and Beyond

AS YOU REACH your seventies, don't fall for the belief that you have to age the way that your mother did. Yes, we all end up with some health problem or another in our seventies (and more likely, we'll juggle several chronic ailments). And the older we get, the more problems we accumulate. But one of the brightest spots in medicine is its ability to help older people control their diseases so they can live longer, higher quality lives. Medicines help, and so do joint replacements, vision surgery, and home adaptations that allow you to remain independent. Best of all, we know that good health habits, especially staying connected to friends and maintaining an exercise routine, can help you squeeze every last drop of juice out of life. And you may still have a lot of juice left: Susan has a seventy-three-year-old friend who just ran the New York City Marathon.

But—and this is a big one—there will be times when you have to balance your independence against your safety. We're talking about driving. You are probably fine to drive in your early seventies, and possibly you will be an excellent driver through your triple digits, but the minute that you or anyone you know starts to question your driving ability, get yourself checked out. Don't rely on the DMV's vision test, which doesn't measure your cognition and judgment. Talk to your doctor, or find out if a local hospital offers driving assessments.

One of the reasons people dread giving up their car keys is that it feels like a one-way ticket to the nursing home. Other limitations, such as hearing loss or frailty, are scary, too, because they threaten to remove you from the people and places you love. The people who handle these challenges most successfully are the ones who acknowledge their limitations while refusing to obediently fade away. They make a mighty effort to foster a large group of friends—both old and new, young and old. Your family is one place to start (grandkids, anyone?), and your place of worship is another. Elder hostels and adult-education programs are also good options that carry the added benefit of keeping your brain sharp.

And be prepared to fight age discrimination in the medical industry! This sword cuts both ways. First, you may have to confront condescension (doctors talk to your kids, not to you) and fatalism (doctors don't tell you about all the potential treatments for a disease). You may have to fight especially hard for adequate pain relief. A 2008 cover story in the *New York Times* cited condescending treatment as such a huge source of stress to older people that it qualifies as a health threat. It also suggested that the most effective way to reduce this stress is to stand up for yourself.

On the other hand, you'll want to be wary of a medical system that is handsomely rewarded each time a Medicare recipient undergoes a procedure—whether or not the patient benefits. More than ever, you'll have to educate yourself about your conditions and which procedures are truly necessary. If you aren't comfortable with computers and the Internet, buddy up with your grandkids or some other young people and have them show you how to research health information in a sensible manner. Demand your right to second and third opinions.

We hope that you will enjoy a chance to relax during these decades—but that you won't take life sitting down. Don't be passive in the face of limitations. Ask for help. Go with your gut. Ali's mother spent the last weeks of her life in a hospice . . . and she had a car pick her up at the hospice building so that she could go run a support group. To the end, she was fully engaged and fully herself. She was gracious, but she didn't go quietly.

And *that* is how to live a Pretty Healthy life.

How to Be Pretty Healthy in Your Seventies and Beyond

- Continue to perform cardiovascular exercise, strength training, and balance work.
- Strengthen your existing relationships and connect with as many new people as you can.

- Eat well. Try to maintain your weight.
- Manage your stress. If your tried-and-true methods of stress relief no longer work, find new ones.
- Don't assume that a chronic disease equals chronic disability. Take the initiative when it comes to learning about resources for adapting to your limitations.
- Consider having your driving skills evaluated regularly.
- If you haven't yet made a living will, do so now.
- Develop your patient-advocacy skills.

At Every Age

HERE'S A WIDELY circulated piece of wisdom that perfectly encapsulates the Pretty Healthy philosophy. No matter how old you are, put this attitude on your to-do list:

"Life's journey is not to arrive at the grave safely in a well-preserved body, but rather to skid in sideways, totally worn out and shouting, 'Holy smokes . . . what a ride!' "

Acknowledgments

When Nancy Snyderman, Elizabeth Browning, and I started LLuminari (now BeWell), we vowed to stay friends no matter what. Through thick and thin we have kept that promise, and the result has been even better than we could have hoped. BeWell, and now this book, are testimony to that bond.

I would like to thank all the wonderful experts of BeWell; I would never have taken on this book without your expertise. Miriam Nelson's input was particularly valuable for the exercise chapter.

Jill Kneerim, my agent, and Heather Jackson, our editor, have been supporters of this collaboration from the beginning.

This book has a much broader point of view thanks to my wonderful coauthor, Ali Domar, and writer Leigh Ann Hirschman. Not only did we have fun on our Tuesday-morning calls, fighting over the data, but we brought our different life perspectives to the topic, making it more reflective of real life.

Finally, I would like to thank the staff of the Dr. Susan Love

Research Foundation, who put up with my extracurricular activities while we work to eradicate breast cancer. Naz Sykes and Dixie Mills are critical to that mission.

—*Susan M. Love*

When I was invited to join the BeWell team in 2001, I was intrigued and honored to be included. But I didn't realize how much fun it would be. Every time we get together, whether for a speaking event, a meal, or a brainstorming session, it is quite simply a blast. I laugh, I learn—just being in the presence of these incredible health experts is amazing. It makes me feel as if I belong to the most popular clique in high school (an experience I missed when I was sixteen). So I would like to thank Elizabeth Browning, Susan Love, and Nancy Snyderman for creating this amazing company and for inviting me to join the ride.

I would also like to thank my coworkers and colleagues—Liz Rodriguez, Derek Larkin, Michael Alper, and everyone at the Domar Center and at Boston IVF—for making my job such a delight. I would not have been able to write this book if it were not for the opportunities you provide to me.

To Chris Tomasino, my agent. You make this an adventure well worth experiencing and your counsel and friendship are so very important to me.

To Heather Jackson, editor extraordinaire: What can I say? I love working with you. You were with us from the get-go, and no question was too minor or stupid. You guided, you prodded, you scheduled a lot of conference calls, and you did it all with humor and affection and wisdom.

To my coauthor, Susan Love: I can't believe we pulled this off!

When two incredibly busy women come at a project from such different backgrounds, you normally have the makings of a battle. But instead, we created a soothing antidote for the women out there whom we both care so much about.

And finally, to Leigh Ann Hirschman: You are a magician. When I told friends and colleagues about our plans for this book, they all said the same thing: "There is no way that a writer will be able to blend the voices of a surgeon and a shrink into one compassionate yet authoritative voice." Yet you proved them all wrong. There is one voice in this book and it so carefully and elegantly combines the way that Susan and I speak and think. Thank you for your skill, your empathy, your friendship, and your dedication to this project.

—*Alice D. Domar*

This project is the result of several supercharged women working together. They include Elizabeth Browning, Jill Kneerim, and Nancy Snyderman, who welcomed me aboard and kept the ship steady; Betsy Amster, whose clear-headedness is a consistent delight; and Heather Jackson, who has the rare ability to zoom in on the details while keeping the big picture in view.

Profound thanks also go to the lovely and levelheaded Heather Proulx and to Crown's crack production staff, including senior production editor Tricia Wygal and copy editor Michelle Daniel.

Ali and Susan, I've loved working with both of you. Your precision, warmth, and tenacity (the good kind) have raised the bar for me. I like to think that I'm a little bit better for having rubbed shoulders with you. I'll miss our weekly calls!

To the BeWell Experts who brainstormed, debated, and shared their stories for this book: Byllye Avery, Christina Economos, Laura

Jana, Loretta LaRoche, Marianne Legato, Miriam Nelson, Hope Ricciotti, Pepper Schwartz, and Nancy Snyderman. I count myself lucky to have been in the same room, and on the phone, with all of you.

I'd also like to thank several women who considerately shared with me their biggest health concerns: Linda Brundage, Ann Cottingham, Andrea Cournoyer, Dee Earl, Sue Hirschman, Betsy Kohn, Kimberly W. Laney, Tina McEntire-Mason, Jody Root, Ginger Rue, and Laura Tiebert. Together, you reminded me that women don't need more scary stories about how their bodies are going to wrack and ruin. They *do* need experts who can help all of us put the health news into a Pretty Healthy perspective. Thanks!

—*Leigh Ann Hirschman*

Selected References

Chapter One. The Myth of Perfect Health

The Alpha-Tocopherol, Beta Carotene Cancer Prevention Study Group, "The Effect of Vitamin E and Beta Carotene on the Incidence of Lung Cancer and Other Cancers in Male Smokers," *New England Journal of Medicine* 15, no. 330 (April 14, 1994): 1029–35.

Nortin M. Hadler, *Worried Sick: A Prescription for Health in an Overtreated America* (Chapel Hill: University of North Carolina Press, 2008).

Michael Pollan, *In Defense of Food: An Eater's Manifesto* (New York: The Penguin Press, 2008).

Chapter Two. Sleep: When Lavender Sachets Don't Work

Scott S. Campbell and Patricia J. Murphy, "The Nature of Spontaneous Sleep Across Adulthood," *Journal of Sleep Research* 16, no. 1 (March 2007).

Richard Ferber, *Solve Your Child's Sleep Problems: New, Revised, and Expanded Edition* (New York: Fireside, 2006).

D. J. Gottlieb, S. Redline, F. J. Nieto, C. M. Baldwin, A. B. Newman, H. E. Resnick, Shawn D. Youngstedt, and Daniel F. Kripke, "Long Sleep and Mortality: Rationale for Sleep Restriction," *Sleep Medicine Reviews* 8 (2004): 159–74.

Daniel F. Kripke, Lawrence Garfinkel, Deborah L. Wingard, Melville R. Klauber, and Matthew R. Marler, "Mortality Associated with Sleep Duration and Insomnia," *Archives of General Psychiatry* 59 (February 2002): 131–35.

Jodi A. Mindell, *Sleeping Through the Night*, rev. ed.: *How Infants, Toddlers, and Their Parents Can Get a Good Night's Sleep* (New York: Collins Living, 2005).

S. R. Patel, N. T. Ayas, M. R. Malhotra, D. P. White, E. S. Schernhammer, F. E. Speizer, M. J. Stampfer, F. B. Hu, "A Prospective Study of Sleep Duration and Mortality Risk in Women," *Sleep* 27, no. 3 (May 1, 2004).

Chapter Three. The Stress Test: How Much Is Too Much?

James A. Blumenthal, Michael A. Babyak, P. Murali Doraiswamy, Lana Watkins, Benson M. Hoffman, Krista A. Barbour, Steve Herman, W. Edward Craighead, Alisha L. Brosse, Robert Waugh, Alan Hinderliter, and Andrew Sherwood, "Exercise and Pharmacotherapy in the Treatment of Major Depressive Disorder," *Psychosomatic Medicine* 69 (2007): 587–96.

Albert Moraska, Terrence Deak, Robert L. Spencer, David Roth, and Monika Fleshner, "Treadmill Running Produces Both Positive and Negative Physiological Adaptations in Sprague-Dawley Rats," *American Journal of Physiology* 48, no. 4 (2000).

Robert M. Sapolsky, *Why Zebras Don't Get Ulcers,* 3rd ed. (New York: Holt, 2004).

Chapter Four. Health Screenings: Do You Really Need a Baseline Mammogram?

Katrina Armstrong, Elizabeth Moye, Sankey Williams, Jesse A. Berlin, and Eileen E. Reynolds, "Screening Mammography in Women 40 to 49 Years of Age: A Systematic Review for the American College of Physicians," *Annals of Internal Medicine* 146 (2007): 516–26.

Joann G. Elmore, Katrina Armstrong, Constance D. Lehman, and Suzanne W. Fletcher, "Screening for Breast Cancer," *Journal of the American Medical Association* 293, no. 10 (2005): 1245–56.

Joann G. Elmore, Mary B. Barton, Victoria M. Moceri, Sarah Polk, Philip J. Arena, and Suzanne W. Fletcher, "Ten-Year Risk of False Positive Screening Mammograms and Clinical Breast Examinations," *New England Journal of Medicine* 338, no. 16 (1998): 1089–96.

U.S. Department of Health and Human Services, Agency for Healthcare Research and Quality, *The Guide to Clinical Preventive Services 2007: Recommendations of the U.S. Preventive Services Task Force* (Washington, D.C.: Agency for Healthcare Research and Quality, 2007).

Chapter Five. It's Not Religion, It's Just Exercise

Andreas Broocks, M.D., Borwin Bandelow, M.D., Gunda Pekrun, M.A., Annette George, M.D., Tim Meyer, M.D., Uwe Bartmann, M.A., Ursula Hillmer-Vogel, M.D., and Eckart Rüther, M.D., "Comparison of Aerobic Exercise, Clomipramine, and Placebo in the Treatment of Panic Disorder," *American Journal of Psychiatry* 155 (May 1998): 603–9.

Martin J. Gibala, Jonathan P. Little, Martin van Essen, Geoffrey P. Wilkin, Kirsten A. Burgomaster, Adeel Safdar, Sandeep Raha, and Mark A. Tarnopolsky, "Short-Term Spring Interval Versus Traditional Endurance Training: Similar Initial Adaptations in Human Skeletal Muscle and Exercise Performance," *Journal of Physiology* 575 (2006): 901–911.

William E. Haskell, I-Min Lee, Russel R. Pate, Kenneth E. Powell, Steven N. Blair, Barry A. Franklin, Caroline A. Macera, Gregory W. Heath, Paul D. Thompson, and Adrian Bauman, "Physical Activity and Public Health: Updated Recommendation for Adults from the American College of Sports Medicine and the American Heart Association," *Circulation* 116, no. 9 (August 1, 2007): 1081–93.

Gina Kolata, "Does Exercise Really Keep Us Healthy?" *New York Times Essentials: Reporter's File,* January 8, 2008, http://health.nytimes.com/ref/health/healthguide/esn-exerciseess.html.

Miriam E. Nelson, W. Jack Rejeski, Steven N. Blair, Pamela W. Duncan, James O. Judge, Abby C. King, Carol A. Macera, and Carmen Castaneda-Sceppa, "Physical Activity and Public Health in Older Adults: Recommendation from the American College of Sports Medicine and the American Heart Association," *Circulation* 116, no. 9 (August 1, 2007): 1094–1105.

Trevor J. Orchard, Marinella Temprosa, Ronald Goldberg, Steven Haffner, Robert Ratner, Santica Marcovina, and Sarah Fowler for the Diabetes Prevention Program, "The Effect of Metformin and Intensive Lifestyle Intervention on the Metabolic Syndrome: The Diabetes Prevention Program Randomized Trial," *Annals of Internal Medicine* 142, no. 19 (2005): 611–19.

Cris A. Slentz, Brian D. Duscha, Johanna L. Johnson, Kevin Ketchum, Lori B. Aiken, Gregory P. Samsa, Joseph A. Houmard, Connie W. Bales, and

William E. Kraus, "Effects of the Amount of Exercise on Body Weight, Body Composition, and Measures of Central Obesity: STRRIDE—A Randomized Controlled Study," *Archives of Internal Medicine* 164, no. 1 (2004): 31–39.

Chapter Six. Eating Well: Beyond Blueberries

Karen I. Bolla, Frank R. Funderburk, and Jean Lud Cadet, "Differential Effects of Cocaine and Cocaine Alcohol on Neurocognitive Performance," *Neurology* 54 (2000): 2285–92.

Lisa Delaney, *Secrets of a Former Fat Girl: How to Lose Two, Four (Or More!) Dress Sizes—and Find Yourself Along the Way* (New York: Plume, 2007).

W. Kalt, Kim Foote, S. A. E. Fillmore, Martha Lyon, T. A. Van Lunen, and K. B. McRae, "Effect of Blueberry Feeding on the Plasma Lipid Levels of Pigs," *British Journal of Nutrition* 100 (2007): 70–78.

Gina Kolata, *Ultimate Fitness: The Quest for Truth About Health and Exercise* (New York: Picador, 2004).

H. Suji, M. G. Larson, and F. J. Venditti, "Impact of Reduced Heart Rate Variability on Risk for Cardiac Events: The Framingham Heart Study," *Circulation* 94 (1996): 2894–95.

Brian Wansink, *Mindless Eating: Why We Eat More Than We Think* (New York: Bantam, 2007).

Walter C. Willett, "The Mediterranean Diet: Science and Practice," *Public Health Nutrition* 9, no. 1A (2006): 105–10.

J. A. Wright, W. F. Velicer, and J. O. Prochaska, "Testing the Predictive Power of the Transtheoretical Model of Behavior Change Applied to Dietary Fat Intake," *Health Education Resources,* April 8, 2008.

National Institutes of Health, "The DASH Diet," http://www.nih.gov/news/pr/apr97/Dash.htm.

Chapter Seven. You, Me, Us: Healthy Relationships

Jennifer Byrd-Craven, David C. Geary, Amanda J. Rose, and Davide Ponzi, "Co-ruminating Increases Stress Hormone Levels in Women," *Hormones and Behavior* 53, no. 3 (2008): 489–92.

N. A. Christakis and J. H. Fowler, "The Spread of Obesity in a Large Social Network Over 32 Years," *New England Journal of Medicine* 357 (2007): 370–79.

E. S. Epel, E. H. Blackburn, J. Lin, F. S. Dhabhar, N. E. Adler, J. D. Morrow, and R. M. Cawthon, "Accelerated Telomere Shortening in Response to Life

Stress," *Proceedings of the National Academy of Sciences* 101, no. 50 (December 14, 2004): 17323–24.

T. O. Harris, G. W. Brown, and R. Robinson, "Befriending as an Intervention for Chronic Depression Among Women in an Inner City: A Randomized Controlled Trial," *British Journal of Psychiatry* 174 (1999): 219–25.

T. O. Harris, G. W. Brown, and R. Robinson, "Role of Fresh-Start Experiences and Baseline Psychosocial Factors in Remission from Depression," *British Journal of Psychiatry* 174 (1999): 225–33.

D. R. Lehman, J. H. Ellard, and C. B. Wortman, "Social Support for the Bereaved: Recipients' and Providers' Perspectives on What Is Helpful," *Journal of Consulting Clinical Psychology* 54 (1986): 438–46.

Amelia R. Turagabeci, Keiko Nakamura, Masashi Kizuki, and Takehito Takano, "Family Structure and Health: How Companionship Acts as a Buffer Against Ill Health," *Health and Quality of Life Outcomes* 5, no. 61 (2007).

Bert N. Uchino, *Social Support and Physical Health: Understanding the Health Consequences of Relationships* (New Haven, Conn.: Yale University Press, 2004).

T. T. Wing and R. W. Jeffery, "Benefits of Recruiting Participants with Friends and Increasing Social Support for Weight Loss and Maintenance," *Journal of Consulting and Clinical Psychology* 67 (1999): 132–38.

Chapter Eight. A Pretty Healthy Life, Decade by Decade

Paolo Boffetta, Joseph K. McLaughlin, Carlo La Vecchia, Robert E. Tarone, Loren Lipworth, and William J. Blot, "False-Positive Results in Cancer Epidemiology: A Plea for Epistemological Modesty," *Journal of the National Cancer Institute* 100 (2008): 888–95.

Steven Woloshin, Lisa M. Schwartz, and H. Gilbert Welch, "The Risk of Death by Age, Sex, and Smoking Status in the United States: Putting Health Risks in Context," *Journal of the National Cancer Institute* 100 (2008): 845–53.

Index

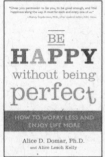
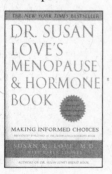